AF480667

SUICIDE
IN JAILS AND PRISONS

SUICIDE

IN JAILS AND PRISONS

PREVENTIVE AND LEGAL PERSPECTIVES

A Guide for Correctional and Mental Health Staff, Experts, and Attorneys

ANASSERIL E. DANIEL, MD

Suicide in Jails and Prisons: Preventive and Legal Perspectives:
A Guide for Correctional and Mental Health Staff, Experts, and Attorneys

For information about this title or to order other books
and/or electronic media, contact the publisher:

Anasseril E. Daniel, MD
www.PrisonSuicideExpertWitness.com
anasserildaniel@gmail.com

ISBNs:
979-8-9852048-2-7 (hardcover)
979-8-9852048-0-3 (softcover)
979-8-9852048-1-0 (eBook)

Printed in the United States of America

Cover and Interior design: 1106 Design

For my family that nurtures my faith in humanity and to my Almamater, National Institute of Mental Health And NeuroSciences (NIMHANS), Bangalore, India, which shaped my interest in psychiatry

TABLE OF CONTENTS

BOOK KEYWORDS

1. Suicide in jails and prisons
2. Custodial suicide
3. Preventing suicide in jails and prisons
4. Lawsuits in jails
5. Suicide-related litigation
6. Deliberate indifference in jails and prisons
7. Medical negligence in jails and prisons
8. Lawsuits against correctional officers
9. Eighth Amendment claims in prisons
10. Suicide screening in jails
11. Suicide risk assessment
12. Experts in suicide-related lawsuits
13. Expert testimony

PREFACE

S*uicide in jails and prisons* is a significant public health issue in the United States and worldwide. It is the leading cause of death in jails and the third leading cause of death in prisons. A lawsuit follows a significant number of suicides.

Suicide in Jails and Prisons: Preventive and Legal Perspectives offers valuable insight into how to prevent suicide and the issues surrounding lawsuits after a suicide or a serious suicide attempt. The book provides guidance, practical tips, standards, and best practices to help stakeholders save lives and avoid lawsuits. It educates the experts who consult and testify in lawsuits and the attorneys who seek such experts. The author, an expert consultant and witness, shares his years of firsthand experience.

Suicide prevention programs in jails and prisons have become a standard in all U.S. jails and prisons. Prevention program stakeholders include members of mental health, medical, correctional, and administrative staff. Each professional plays a unique role in preventing suicide and must take specific risk identification and preventive intervention steps.

Psychiatrists, psychologists, mental health professionals, and correctional officers working in jails and prisons may become subjects of a lawsuit after an inmate under their care commits suicide. Such lawsuits claim medical malpractice and deliberate indifference by the clinicians and jail personnel. Mental health professionals, correctional officers, and administrators should know the best practices of their profession. They must also be proficient in its policies, procedures, and risk management strategies.

The readers of this book will gain knowledge in:

1. inmate suicide risk identification;
2. suicide risk assessment;
3. best practices in suicide prevention;
4. preventive steps to save lives;
5. legal principles of malpractice and deliberate indifference lawsuits;
6. how to be an effective expert witness; and
7. how to select an expert consultant and/or a witness.

For the expert retained by an attorney, this book provides a road map for conducting an objective analysis to support or refute a claim. For an attorney trying to hire an expert, the book offers guidance and strategies on whether to try a case or settle it. Also, the book provides insights for families who have lost loved ones to suicide.

The book offers these special features:

1. It gives special emphasis to correctional officers' role in prevention.
2. It combines prevention and legal aspects of suicide.
3. It describes a methodology for experts to analyze legal claims.

4. Through case histories, the book shows readers what could go wrong in the management of suicidal inmates and the legal process, and it offers possible solutions.

Suicide in Jails and Prisons: Preventive and Legal Perspectives will be a useful guide for correctional psychiatrists, psychologists, clinicians, nurses, officers, administrators, experts, and attorneys.

FOREWORD

Save your brain cells for the emergencies.

Regardless of whether I am speaking to nurses working in jails or medical students in class, I often use this hyperbolic statement to encourage colleagues to make routine what can be made routine. Routine steps, routine procedures, and routine evidence-based screening tools save mental energy and lives—particularly when practicing medicine in high-risk environments. Jails, prisons, and detention centers are such environments.

When people are incarcerated, particularly in their early hours and days of confinement, they are not at their best. They have been arrested. They have had their autonomy and communication limited. They may have an undiagnosed or undertreated chronic medical illness, mental illness, or substance use disorder. They have new clothes, new roommates, a new diet, and a new schedule. They are now living in environments that are loud and bright and uncomfortable. They may be withdrawing from a psychoactive substance or therapeutic medication. And they may have committed a crime.

All these factors contribute to the high rates of suicide in U.S. correctional and detention facilities.

The overlay of COVID-19, the opioid overdose epidemic, and the frank exploration of institutional racism have created deep disruption throughout communities and institutions in the U.S. since early 2020. Few systems demonstrate the brokenness of our institutions through these crises as does the U.S. criminal justice system.

In recent years, sentencing and prison reform were acted on with bipartisan support—at least in 2018 at a federal level with the First Step Act. This legislation reflects the almost universal recognition that significant reform is long overdue. Then, in 2020, as COVID-19 started spreading throughout the country, the health and well-being of people incarcerated in jails, prisons, and detention centers, typically overlooked populations in the United States, became a featured topic in public health, legal forums, and the media.

While this recognition for system change is laudable, it does not address the immediate concern of those now incarcerated. People currently detained in jails, prisons, and detention centers have emergent, urgent, and chronic conditions that require medical care. One of the most pressing needs is mental health care, which includes addressing suicidality among detainees.

The factors mentioned above, coupled with the lack of access to health care of many of those detainees from minority and under-resourced communities prior to incarceration, create an environment of elevated stressors among those typically already experiencing mental illness and distress. Moreover, the workforce available to evaluate, diagnose, and treat these individuals remains underdeveloped and undertrained.

That is exactly why Dr. A.E. Daniel's text is needed in this field. Health-care providers in correctional settings need training and resources to successfully provide the best clinical advice to patients, medical colleagues, and correctional colleagues, as well as to create standards, and ultimately, mitigate the risk of suicide in correctional settings.

As a faculty physician at Saint Louis University in Missouri, my clinical practice has focused on correctional health care, homeless health care, and addiction medicine. Board-certified in family medicine and in addiction medicine, I was the medical director and lead physician for the St. Louis County Jail and Juvenile Detention Center for over fifteen years. I recently completed my first anniversary as medical director for juvenile detention for the 22nd Circuit Court in the City of St. Louis. In recent years, I have served as a subject matter expert—for both plaintiffs and defendants—in suits related to detainee deaths, detention conditions, and, most recently, the response of jails to mitigate the risks associated with COVID-19 for detainees.

A consistent theme in my work has been the need to advance the field of correctional health care with concrete, evidence-based clinical tools to mitigate harm, promote health, and protect those who do this critical, but often litigious work.

I was introduced to Dr. Daniel by Percy Menzies, president of Assisted Recovery Centers of America (ARCA). Dr. Dan, as Percy refers to him, was a "godsend" to ARCA in its early years. Percy struggled to find physicians who would join him in his pioneering work to create a treatment model for substance use disorders that was patient-centered, humane, and allowed a person to recover in-place/at-home whenever possible. Dr. Daniel provided the physician care necessary for this team-based approach to care, and his contribution gave Percy the capacity and the space to build one of the largest practices in the Midwest that brings in-person and telehealth services to people throughout Missouri.

Percy's expectation that we would see eye to eye on treatment philosophy and patient care was confirmed with our first phone call last year. Dr. Daniel and I shared stories about our work and our frustration about the lack of standardization in our fields of practice. This lack of standardization puts both detainees and correctional officers at risk.

Society expects a great deal from these custodial professionals, and clear guidelines, including training schedules and professional development around mental illness and suicide, helps them work effectively and consistently. I eagerly agreed when Dr. Daniel asked me to review and edit his text chapters as he was writing them.

In time, as the book developed, he asked me to contribute some of the medication guidelines I had developed for substance use disorders at the St. Louis County Jail, which were further refined at ARCA. Then he invited me to undertake a new challenge—writing a foreword for his text.

Dr. Daniel has an impressive career as a psychiatrist who has practiced in a variety of high-intensity settings. He practiced for several years in the Missouri Department of Corrections, where he also served as the Director of Psychiatric Services. His scholarship is prolific—from authorship to editing to updating guidelines on suicide prevention with the World Health Organization. He is a clinician and scholar who can do the work and then translate his experience for others. His current work as an expert witness is informed by his roles as a psychiatrist, medical director, and administrator. He is passionate about sharing what he has learned and practiced in advancing the field of health care for the incarcerated, so that all stakeholders can have the safest, healthiest outcome possible.

I have invested many hours reviewing and discussing this text with Dr. Daniel. As many hours as I have spent, I see as many applications as possible in this text. This text can be a much-needed resource for correctional physicians and health team members. It can be a starting point for specific guidelines and standards of care. It can be a training tool for psychiatric residents and primary care residents interested in the field. And law students can use the book as a primer for standards of care for clients and for advocacy work.

This text has no peers in the field of exploring and mitigating risks of suicide in correctional settings. It promotes the common good of all stakeholders, since it gathers and clarifies practices and court rulings pertaining to the care of detainees at risk of suicide.

As Maya Angelou famously stated, "Do the best you can until you know better. Then, when you know better, do better." Dr. Daniel's work gives us the tools to do better.

—Fred Rottnek, MD, MAHCM
Professor and Director of Community Medicine,
Program Director, Addiction Medicine Fellowship,
Department of Family and Community Medicine
Saint Louis University School of Medicine

Professor, Center for Health Law Studies, Saint Louis University School of Law

Professor, Doisy College of Health Sciences, Physician Assistant Program

SLUCare Academic Pavilion, 1008 South Spring Ave., St. Louis, Missouri, 63110

INTRODUCTION

Suicide in jails and prisons is a significant public health issue in the United States and worldwide. It is the leading cause of death in jails and the third leading cause of death in prisons. What's more, lawsuits often follow suicides.

Suicide prevention programs are now standard in all U.S. jails and prisons. Stakeholders of these prevention programs include each facility's mental health, medical, correctional, and administrative staff. Each of these professionals takes specific steps in risk identification and preventive intervention.

Typically, mental health and medical staff perform suicide risk assessment. To that extent, the clinicians must identify risk factors, perform suicide risk assessment, and monitor and treat an at-risk inmate by adhering to best practices. In addition to their traditional safety and security responsibilities, correctional officers are the eyes and ears of suicide prevention programs.

During my work as an administrator and psychiatrist in the Missouri Department of Corrections and Boone County Jail, I became intimately familiar with how mental health professionals, policymakers, and correctional officers attempt to fulfill their unique roles in preventing inmates from taking their lives. My research on suicide, my clinical experience of working with potentially suicidal inmates, with staff training, and with expert consultations on suicide-related litigation during the last two decades have shaped my thinking in developing a few, simple-to-follow steps to make every stakeholder's job easier and their prevention efforts more effective. In that sense, this book reflects my passionate commitment to prevent suicides in jails and prisons and train the professionals involved. Thus, the book reflects my firm conviction that most suicides in jails and prisons are preventable.

The book has two parts:

PART I

In the first five chapters, I discuss the characteristics of inmates who attempt suicide, the methods they use, theories explaining the phenomenon of suicide, and the relationship of suicide to mental illness, substance abuse, and institutional risk factors, along with the best practices of suicide risk assessment. Additionally, I provide guidelines, standards, and practical tips for psychiatrists, psychologists, other mental health professionals, and correctional officers on risk iden-tification, assessment, and interventions to prevent suicides and save lives.

IN PART II

In the next six chapters, I discuss the common causes of law-suits related to suicide in jails and prisons, legal liability risk management strategies, expert analysis methodology, report writing, deposition strategies, and attorneys' perspectives on experts. I also include nine case histories outlining legal course of action.

The estate or the survivors of the deceased file a variety of lawsuits against professionals, the facilities, and the government for negligence, medical malpractice, ADA-based claims, and what is known as "deliberate indifference," a violation of the deceased's constitutional rights. I discuss legal components of deliberate indifference, what constitutes a serious medical need, and the standards of proof required for such a claim. Stakeholders can use various legal liability risk management strategies to avoid lawsuits.

A typical lawsuit against a mental health professional aims to establish either malpractice (medical negligence), a deliberate indifference claim, or both. Nonadherence by a clinician to the standard of care can lead to a medical negligence claim. Cities, counties, and states have paid millions in settlement for legal claims involving preventable suicides. Violation of an inmate's constitutional rights by clinicians, correctional officers, and administration can lead to a deliberate indifference claim, often referred to as a §1983 claim.

A lawsuit is won or lost by presenting reliable evidence to a judge or a jury. An expert witness plays a crucial role in the lawsuit's outcome because the subject matter is beyond the realm of common knowledge judges and jurors are presumed to bring to trial. Experts in such cases may include psychiatrists, jail and prison policy developers, nurses with correctional experience, jail/prison administrators, and anyone with specialized education, skill, knowledge, experience, and expertise in the correctional field. Experts with such qualifications are in high demand by the legal system.

There is no standard methodology to analyze the claims of civil rights violations involving suicide or attempted suicide.

This book, however, provides a road map to help experts perform a well-reasoned analysis to objectively support or refute such claims. A reliable methodology will be useful to serve the ends of justice.

An expert must perform objective analysis of care documents and policies and procedures to determine if a malpractice or deliberate indifference claim is meritorious. As per Federal Rules of Civil Procedure 26, commonly known as Rule 26, an expert is required to submit a report of his/her analysis. The expert must prepare a report outlining all opinions in a manner that reflects a reliable methodology so that the expert can present and defend those opinions during deposition and trial.

Based on my consults in more than seventy-five lawsuits in the U.S., I provide advice and guidelines on how to be an effective expert witness and how to give an excellent deposition. I further discuss commonly raised questions and topics that become the subject of inquiry during a deposition in a suicide-related lawsuit.

For attorneys, I outline characteristics of a credible expert. After the report production and deposition, an attorney may consider settling the case or proceeding with a trial. Finally, the judicial proceedings and the timeline of a docket order are outlined.

Case studies from expert consultations illustrate the salient points of case analysis and judicial outcome.

The book combines the preventive and legal aspects of suicide in jails and prisons. It is my sincere hope that it will be a useful guide for mental health and medical providers, correctional officers, and jail and prison administrators who strive to minimize suicides in their facilities and avoid legal liability claims. For attorneys who seek experts to assist them in laying out their cases with expert consultants and witnesses, the book will provide valuable direction and assistance.

In the Appendix, I outline a typical outline to train the staff, provide an easy-to-follow checklist for administrators, mental health staff, and correctional officers, and alcohol and opiate detoxification protocols. In addition, I include several prominent attorneys' perspectives on selection of experts.

—Anasseril E. Daniel, MD

PART I

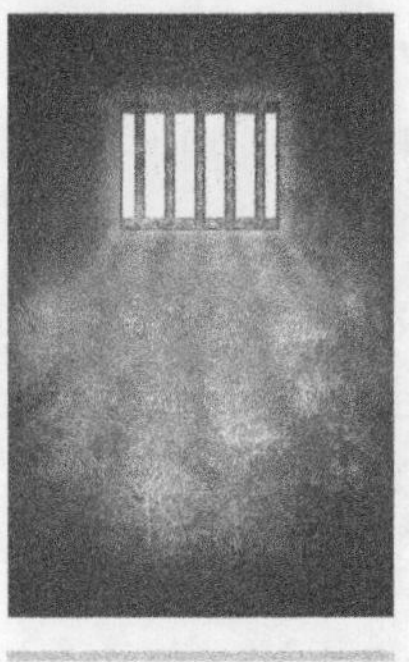

CHAPTER 1

SUICIDAL IDEATION, ATTEMPTS, METHODS, AND THEORIES

*(Who, what, how, and why of suicide
attempts and suicide)*

DEFINITIONS

Suicidal ideation is defined as the verbal expression of thoughts of ending one's life. A *suicide attempt* depicts a behavior to end one's life that failed. *Suicidal gesture* is an act simulating an attempted suicide, usually designed to attract attention, but inadequately planned. A person with a *suicidal tendency* has a history of suicidal ideation and has made suicide attempts.

A "suicide alert" refers to a status placed on an inmate after review of information and evidence of suicidal behavior by the appropriate professional.

3

Suicide observation is an essential activity by the staff to observe an inmate at risk for suicide with the purpose of preventing any self-destructive act. A detainee or an inmate may be placed on suicide observation by any member of the staff, including custody, medical, or mental health personnel. Suicide observation can be discontinued only by a duly credentialed mental health professional.

The term *suicide watch* is sometimes used interchangeably with *suicide observation* for an intense monitoring process to ensure that an inmate cannot attempt suicide. An inmate to be watched will be placed in a suicide observation cell, which is a designated cell devoid of any materials or anchor points on which to hang.

SUICIDAL IDEATION

A suicidal thought accompanied by intent and a plan to self-harm, with access to means such as a weapon, a noose, or drugs may result in suicidal death. Hence, ideation is the first link in a sequence of events culminating in suicide. Next in the continuum of risk is the inmate having access to the means to accomplish the suicide.

The combination of ideation, accessibility to means, and having a plan, represents an imminent suicide risk.

The intent and plan may not always be evident except by suicide notes, change in behaviors (e.g., giving away possessions, withdrawal from contact with other inmates and family), and symptoms (e.g., anxiety, depression, feelings of hopelessness, agitation, irritability, impulsivity, and insomnia). Sometimes, the intent may be suspect in certain inmates who want to manipulate the officers or disrupt the system milieu. Some inmates may merely have thoughts or a wish not to be alive, with no apparent intent to kill themselves. Such thoughts may be intermittent and transient.

Many inmates who entertain current suicidal ideation have a history of past suicide attempts. Suicidal ideation may also predict future suicide attempts; however, it does not necessarily predict completed suicide.

An understanding of the unique characteristics of suicidal ideation is essential to evaluate inmate suicide risk. How inmates communicate suicidal ideation differs significantly from those in the public. Very often, inmates at risk conceal their thoughts. Only 40% of the inmates with suicidal ideation disclose them to others, primarily because the correctional setting does not foster self-disclosure, though many who kill themselves leave suicidal notes.[1] The low percentage of inmates who report suicide ideation is in stark contrast with psychiatric outpatients who commit suicide. Almost 90% of outpatients communicate their thoughts to harm themselves to their therapists.[2]

Correctional officers are the least favored recipients of inmate self-disclosure of suicidal ideation or notes. More commonly, inmates communicate their death wish to family members, mental health professionals, and judges.

Inmates often deny their true intent before the suicide, fearful that they will be stripped of their clothes and placed in a suicide observation cell. Most inmates prefer their own cell to a suicide observation cell. They even deny the suicidal thoughts when directly asked to avoid placement in a suicide-resistant smock.

Only half of inmates may tell the staff about their suicidal ideation immediately before they take their lives.[3]

Staff members commonly take the denial of suicidal ideation at face value. However, careful observation of inmate behaviors and emotional states will yield clues to their true intent. Often, inmates are more comfortable expressing suicidal thoughts to other inmates, who may be reluctant to disclose such information to officers. The inmates may occasionally disclose their pain and traumatic memories and how they impact their functioning to mental health staff. In most cases, inmate suicides are preventable, so it is important to recognize the warning signs of impending suicide.

SUICIDE ATTEMPTS

It is often tempting to prejudge a suicide attempt as manipulative when offenders are antisocial and engage in repeat gestures. However, a suicide attempt is a sentinel event requiring immediate clinical and administrative intervention and tracking. All suicide attempts should be taken seriously.

Suicide attempters generally conform to a typical profile

The attempters (as opposed to those who complete suicide) are generally younger (mid-twenties), have previously attempted suicide, have a history of psychiatric treatment, and are addicted to opiates or other substances.[4] Most repeat attempters slash their wrists, as opposed to hanging or overdosing on medication, both common among completers.[5] Many show frustration with their arrest and incarceration but are not committed to dying.[6] Although women may attempt suicide more often than men, men are three to four times more successful in completing suicide than women.[7]

Prior suicide attempts increase the risk of suicide deaths
Retrospective studies have shown that 33% to 66% of prison suicides were preceded by previous attempts or gestures.[8, 9, 10, 11, and 12] In general, at least half of individuals attempt suicide before the completed act, and half of those who have tried have done so on more than one occasion.

Inmates may exhibit non-lethal and lethal means of self-harm. Non-lethal means include slashing, self-cutting, and headbanging. Some researchers contend that non-lethal and lethal attempters are fundamentally different[13] in their motivation. Others view all self-harm acts on a continuum since the motivation for self-injurious behavior is the same for both attempters and completers. [14]

Some inmates attempt suicide with no intention of completing the suicidal act, while others intensify their lethal methods until achieving death. Inmates may use suicidal statements as a game to get attention. Because it is hard to distinguish between gaming and genuine ideation, officers must treat all suicidal behaviors or statements as legitimate.

The author studied the profile of offenders who seriously attempted suicide in a large state correctional system for thirty months.[15] The subjects were classified into two groups: 1) Lethal attempters who attempted suicide using hanging and overdose; 2) Nonlethal attempters who used methods such as slashing, cutting, etc. It was hypothesized that the suicide attempters who resort to potentially lethal means such as hanging and overdose were significantly different from the nonlethal attempters who used slashing, cutting, and head-banging. The cohort of lethal attempters was then compared with a cohort of inmates who completed suicide (suicide completers) from an earlier study from the same system on select variables.[1]

Data from the study indicate that serious attempters were mostly White males who had committed property crimes, rather than crimes against people, and short-term convicts (sentence <10 years). Seventy-eight percent had a psychiatric diagnosis, of which depressive disorder of mild to moderate severity was most common. Concerning symptoms, depression, feelings of hopelessness, anxiety, and surprisingly, hallucinations, were the most common symptoms before the suicide attempt. Some type of psychosocial stressor influenced 69% of attempters. The majority (74%) had a cellmate at the time of the attempt. Almost 50% were housed in maximum security facilities. Most of these inmates were not on suicide watch at the time of the attempt; however, twenty-five inmates were either on watch at the time of the attempt or had recently been taken off suicide watch. The most common method for a suicide attempt was overdosing on medication or cutting the wrists. Eleven inmates made false claims concerning their suicide attempts, (i.e., they said they had attempted suicide by overdose when, in fact, no drugs had been ingested.) A significant proportion (48%) chose potentially lethal methods such as attempted hanging and overdose. These lethal attempters tend to be genuine in their intent, and they had many features common to those who committed suicide.

The near-lethal group, when compared with a cohort of thirty-seven inmates[1] who committed suicide, showed no significant differences in gender, race, age, crime type, diagnosis, prior or current psychiatric care, and substance abuse. However, symptoms such as delusions, hallucinations, impulsivity, guilt feelings, being subjected to conflicts, ridicule, and rape were more common in the completers. Furthermore, completers tended to have more new convictions, medical conditions, psychosocial stressors and prior suicidal behaviors, and were likely to be held in single cells. Hanging and medication overdose was more common among the lethal attempters.

The ratio of all suicide attempters to completers (112 versus 4) during the 30 months, was 28:1. The rate rises to 13:1 when calculated as the proportion of lethal attempters to completers. This ratio indicates that the risk of fatality is higher among those who used methods such as attempted hanging and overdose.

The previous failed use of a lethal suicide attempt such as attempted hanging or overdose is a significant predictor of successful suicide.

Failed lethal suicide attempts and deficiencies in risk assessment are correlated with high rates of future suicide. Therefore, a comprehensive suicide risk assessment is an important tool in identifying high-risk inmates. Placing failed lethal suicide attempters in the risk management category decreases the chance of suicide. In some jails and prisons, a serious/lethal suicide attempter is tagged for daily intervention by mental health staff and observation by the officers until the inmate's suicide risk no longer exists.

Marzano et al.[16] noted that there is a strong association between near-lethal self-harm and mental disorders, which underscores the importance of screening for mental disorder and suicidality, at the earliest point in the criminal justice pathway.

A past failed near-lethal suicide attempt is associated with high suicide intent.[1, 16] Inmates entering the system with this history will likely act on their intent in the early stages of incarceration, thus indicating a strong need for systematic suicide screening at reception into jails or prisons.

MANIPULATIVE SUICIDE ATTEMPTS

Some inmates use suicidal behavior to control the environment. They are viewed as manipulative. This is true for inmates who have a history of rule breaking and conduct violations. Some may have antisocial personality or borderline personality disorder and may find it difficult to adjust to an overly controlled environment such as maximum-security units and/or administrative segregation.

Intent and manipulativeness may co-exist in an individual

A high degree of intent and manipulative behavior may co-exist, particularly in those who want to have a change in their environment such as transfer out of highly regimented environment.

If the correctional staff believes an inmate is trying to manipulate the environment, they may not take his/her self injurious behaviors seriously by labeling them as suicide gestures. If an inmate's self-injurious behavior is described as a suicide gesture, it does not convey the inmate's true intent. American Psychiatric Association has "retired" the term suicide gesture in clinical practice.[30] Suicide attempts, whatever their motivation, can result in death, even if this was not the original intent.[17] Due to the limited availability of methods in a correctional environment, they may choose the most lethal method, such as hanging, even if they do not wish to die without knowing the dangerousness of the method.[18] In other words, a manipulative attempter may unwittingly choose the most lethal method.

METHODS OF SUICIDE

Hanging

Approximately 90% of suicides in jails and prisons are completed by hanging. This is because the inmates don't have access to firearms, a preferred means in the community.

Hanging as a method of suicide is defined as an intentional act of suspending one's body from a height with a noose tied around the neck from an anchor point. It can also occur from jumping from a height with a ligature around the neck from an anchor point. The method is simple and requires fewer resources (like a firearm or drugs). An inmate can hang with the materials and resources already available in a detention cell or supplied to him/her during their stay.

Hanging requires an anchor point. In many cells, anchor points are readily available. If they are not, an inmate may use other means, such as commodes or toilets, as anchor points. Commonly used anchor points in a cell include windowsills, ventilation grates, light fixtures, upper bunks, hooks, and doorknobs.

Bedsheets may be torn to create a rope. Pieces of clothing, telephone cords, electric cords, shoelaces, and very occasionally, ropes made of toilet paper made firm by rice paste, may be used to create a noose.

Even if an inmate is placed in a suicide-resistant cell with no working electric outlets, recessed lighting, fixed bed, anchor points, or other object that can be converted into a sharp object or a hook, grate, or knob, he/she will find ingenious ways to hang. For instance, one inmate tore a bedsheet and tied it loosely around the base of the toilet in his cell. Then he crawled under the toilet, placed his head through the "noose" around the toilet, and pulled himself away, leaving him unconscious. He died shortly thereafter.

Mechanism of death by hanging

The mortality rate from hanging is exceptionally high compared with other self-harm methods. Gunnell et al. reported that hanging ends in death at least 70% of the time.[19] Those who survive a hanging may end up with medical complications such as quadriplegia or a vegetative state due to prolonged brain anoxia.

Studies of the pathophysiology of death by hanging show that there are four potential mechanisms of death: 1. respiratory asphyxia; 2. interruption of cerebral blood flow due to the occlusion of vessels in the neck, causing cerebral anoxia; 3. cardiac inhibition secondary to nerve stimulation[20]; and 4. snapping of the vertebra at C2 or C3 level, mostly seen in judicial hanging where there is a long drop. (Long drops are infrequent in suicide by hanging in a jail setting.)

Generally, brain damage occurs in 3 to 5 minutes and death in 5 to 7 minutes.

The time it takes a person to die depends on whether by a short or long drop and on the person's circulatory status. It may take longer to lose consciousness when a young person with relatively healthy carotid vessels lays down with the rope tied to the door handle (a short drop). In some situations, it may take up to half an hour before total death occurs by asphyxiation. In a long drop, where there is snapping of C2 or C3 or blocking off carotid arteries, death may happen in few seconds or instantaneously.

An understanding of the time it takes for a person to die from hanging is critical from a preventive programmatic perspective. As noted above, death usually occurs in 5 to 7 minutes in most cases of suicide in a cell. Typically, officers perform cell checks every 30 minutes in the general population. Inmates on suicide watch are checked every 15 minutes. Such intervals allow enough time for those intent on killing themselves to plan and carry out hanging without raising the alarm from officers or sleeping cellmates. I know of numerous incidents where death from hanging occurred in between checks.

Overdose

The second most common method of suicide is by ingestion of large quantities of prescription medications with lethal potential. Such medications may include tricyclic antidepressants such as imipramine or amitriptyline. The usual lethal dose of imipramine is about 30 pills of 100 mg each. Some may ingest a combination of prescription medications and illegal drugs. In most jails and prisons, the psychotropic medications are administered on a "watch take" (self-administered, supervised by a nurse) basis. However, many who overdose may hoard enough pills by "cheeking." Some jails allow "keep on person" non-psychiatric medications such as nitroglycerine, blood pressure medications, antibiotics, anti-allergic agents, and common over-the-counter medications. An inmate committed suicide with verapamil, an antihypertensive, ingesting more than 3000 mg (personal knowledge).

Uncommon methods of suicide

1. Jumping from a top tier or some high location in the jail
2. Self-strangulation/self-suffocation by wrapping a garbage bag over the neck and tightening it, causing cerebral anoxia
3. Head smashing by running at high speed into a concrete wall
4. Hunger strike
5. Self-immolation
6. Jumping in front of a moving vehicle during furlough
7. Suicide masquerading as homicide
8. Having someone kill the victim or allowing oneself to be victimized
9. Chewing on arm and bleeding to death
10. Self-cutting on the jugular vein or cubital artery
11. Stuffing a T-shirt into throat and suffocating
12. Drinking cleaning fluid from a housekeeper's cart

THEORIES OF CUSTODIAL SUICIDE

In custodial settings, inmates commit suicide due to a complex interaction of psychiatric, biological, genetic, and psychosocial factors, including institutional stress. Inmates are housed in a controlled setting where they form an artificial, but loosely integrated society. Inmates come from different backgrounds, face pretrial detention, or serve variable sentences, and have different levels of coping skills and resources. Additionally, they must comply with institutional restrictions, supervision, and rules, which some find unacceptable and intimidating. They may rebel against these rules, adding undue stress. Those placed in administrative segregation and maximum-security prisons face rigid environment and sensory deprivation. These settings make a difference in the life and psychological status of the inmates, compared with those in the rest of the community.

Many questions arise in studying the custodial suicide. What theories and hypotheses best explain it? What makes an inmate take his or her life? Is an inmate's suicide foreseeable? Are all suicides in correctional setting preventable? While one death is not acceptable from a moral, ethical, or medical standpoint, what is an acceptable rate of suicide in jail or prison?

Classical theories of suicide include Durkheim's social integration, Shneidman's "psychache,"[21] Freud's death instinct, Joiner's Interpersonal-Psychological theory,[22] and some lesser-known constructs, such as Steve Taylor's power of purpose.[23] Certain theories, such as Seligman's theory of learned helplessness[24] and Beck's theory of hopelessness,[25] may explain the mental state of the inmate at the time of suicide, but do not fully explain why an inmate commits suicide.

These theories and constructs have important implications for the development of therapeutic and preventive intervention, but none solely explain the cause of suicide in a custodial setting. However, examining these theories is worth the pursuit.

French sociologist Emile Durkheim (1858–1917) put forth the most widely accepted theory of suicide. His theory is based on a person's integration into society. An integrated society is created when people's beliefs, values, and shared customs and traditions bind them together. According to Durkheim, suicide is inversely related to how well a person has integrated into society.

Durkheim classified suicide into four types: egoistic, anomic, fatalistic, and altruistic.

The egoistic type best fits most suicides in jails and prisons, because many inmates are disenfranchised and alienated from society. Unable to adjust to family and society, they have only limited connections in their lives.

Anomic suicide involves individuals whose situation has changed so dramatically that norms are no longer relevant to them. This type of suicide occurs among those whose status has changed drastically after the arrest, especially those who held high social status before their arrest.

Fatalistic suicide occurs among inmates in maximum security units and administrative segregation, where they find themselves trapped with feelings of "no way out"—such as a life sentence with no possibility of parole.

Altruistic suicide, found in those who sacrifice their own lives for a higher purpose to serve a group hardly ever occurs in a controlled setting like a jail or prison.

Thomas Joiner [2005][22] proposed that "thwarted belongingness" and being a burden on others are the basis of self-harm. His theory states that thwarted belongingness is a painful mental state when a person's fundamental need for connectedness is unmet, resulting in the person feeling he/she is an undue burden to others. Such a mental state may be a significant factor for many inmates. A few serious almost lethal attempts and completed suicides occur immediately after divorce papers are filed, or a rejection letter from a loved one is received.

Sigmund Freud's theory is based on "Thanatos"—the death instinct. Some inmates may entertain a death wish, which may or may not be obvious to others. Typically, middle-aged, chronically depressed inmates detained for a minor offense express their wish to die and act out impulsively. They are unlikely to have a history of prior suicide attempt or active suicidal ideation.

A better understood theory from a pragmatic perspective is that of Erik Erikson, who postulated that a person commits suicide when overwhelming feelings of guilt exceed the ability to cope.[26] Many first-time detainees fall into this category due to overwhelming guilt for their impulsive criminal behavior and lack of coping skills to adjust to a life behind bars. A female homicidal offender, particularly a battered spouse or partner who acted in self-defense vis-a-vis persistent abuse by her husband or partner, may find herself engaging in suicidal behaviors out of guilt, both because of her actions and her lack of emotional coping resources.

Edwin Shneidman's "psychache" theory of suicide is based on psychological and emotional pain that reaches intolerable intensity.

Lyn Abramson et al.[27, 23] proposed in 2000 that feelings of hopelessness accounted for suicidal ideation and behavior. She further noted that suicidality is the core symptom of hopelessness and depression. Aaron T. Beck elaborated the association among depression, hopelessness, and suicidality. Beck found that feelings of hopelessness are the predominant mental state in those who commit suicide almost 90% of the time.

Bonner and Rich (1990)[28] studied a stress-psychosocial vulnerability model of suicidal ideation and behavior in a jail population. They administered psychological measures of social alienation, cognitive distortions, adaptive resources, situational (jail environment) stress, depression, hopelessness, and suicide ideation in 146 male inmates at a county jail facility. They found that combination of low reasons for living, irrational beliefs, jail stress, and loneliness best explained suicidal intent.

Thus, various theories and postulates suggest that depression, hopelessness, a feeling of being trapped (helplessness), lack of connectedness, and guilt are the predominant mental state(s) at the time of a suicidal act. Yet not all inmates who experience such states take their lives. The most plausible and easily understood explanation of custodial suicide incorporates the key elements of Durkheim's social integration model and Beck's theory of depression and hopelessness.

Inmate risk factors for suicide attempts and completed suicides have been identified in multiple studies.[1, 3, 17] These risk factors are supported by research and are well established. One framework for understanding suicide risk involves identifying both the static risk factors (those that are chronic, demographic, or relatively unchanging during a person's lifetime) and the dynamic risk factors (those that are short-term, acute, and have to do with a person's current state of mind or situation). Individuals with significant static risk factors may always be at an elevated risk for suicide, but when they experience additional dynamic (situational and sometimes temporary) risk factors, a critical mental state arises.

As the name suggests, static factors are non-variable. They include ages over fifty-five, male sex, Caucasian, severe mental disorder, substance abuse, maximum security detention, pre-trial status, past suicide attempt, and similar non-changeable factors.

The commonly observed dynamic factors include loss of a loved one, impending divorce (which may be related to the arrest and potential criminal prosecution), loss of custody of children, an unusually long sentence, an unexpected additional charge or sentence, placement in a maximum-security unit, loss of dignity and standing in the community, and other, similar psychosocial stressors. Other dynamic factors include (in no specific order): alcohol intoxication and withdrawal; and opioid/heroin withdrawal, mainly when there is minimal recognition of withdrawal symptoms or inadequate treatment. Although these are high-risk factors, not all inmates who have all or some of them kill themselves. Correlation is not necessarily causation, though risk factors that occur in clusters increase the likelihood of suicide. Not any single factor (with the probable exception of a prior near-lethal suicide attempt) increases the risk. Risk factors must occur in the context of a pathogenic mental state in an individual prone to impulsive acting out.

There is a common pathway to inmate suicide

When static factors individually or collectively interact with dynamic factors in an inmate's life, given the opportunity and the means, he or she takes his/her life. The dynamic factors, events, or circumstances act as immediate precipitants of the self-destructive act. Almost always, an event or circumstance occurs in an inmate's life that acts as a catalyst. Most suicides are the result of impulsive decision-making. When feelings of hopelessness occur in the context of narrowing prospects accompanied by loss of options for coping, suicide vulnerability reaches its peak.

The critical mental state of hopelessness in the context of narrowing options and coping, coupled with behavior traits such as impulsivity, agitation, and tension are observed among those acutely and imminently suicidal. Impulsivity and aggression are highly correlated with suicidal behavior across psychiatric samples and non-psychiatric populations. Impulsivity and aggression are related, but the nature of this relationship remains unclear, though many inmates are both impulsive and aggressive.[29]

CONCLUSION

A clear understanding of the who, what, how, and why of suicides in jails and prisons enhances strategies the stakeholders must take to save lives. Many times, providers are at a loss as to how to identify an inmate at risk and provide appropriate interventional help. Officials' high degree of suspicion of suicidality of inmates and timely and proper completion of screening procedures, risk assessment, and compliance with jail/prison policy and procedures will go a long way to preventing suicides (to be discussed in the subsequent chapters).

AN INMATE SUICIDE NOTE

The following excerpt from a suicide note found in the cell of a twenty-five-year-old inmate, who hanged himself illustrates his agony, pain, and feelings of hopelessness.

(It is unclear whether he copied the piece from a book)

He wrote:

I suffer from a blight of banality and crippling mental stagnation so vexing, so disinheriting, that I actually think of death as my only creative work awaiting me. What is this sudden affliction of the mind? This cancer that has so abruptly and mercilessly eviscerated my creative ability? I hate myself: I loathe my inane mind. I am a boorish lout. A venerable waste of precious oxygen and an incompetent, inept, unskilled failure of biology leeching off the creative fruit of my intelligence. I am a bungle of life, a butcher of tasks, a blunder, and flounder; a bumbler and am only maladroit and unimaginative that even a wall covered in freshly applied white paint piques more interest in passers-by. I am so inexpert and incapable of coloring any aspect of my existence that nature disdains me. I am a grave disappointment to her. I feel so deeply that I have been cursed.

REFERENCES

1. Daniel, AE and Fleming, J. *Suicides in a State Correctional System 1992–2002, a Review.* Journal of Correctional Health Care 12: [1] (2006): 24–35

2. Earle, KA, Forquer, SL, Volo, AM and McDonnell, PM. *Characteristics of Outpatient Suicides.* Hospital and Community Psychiatry 45 (2) (1994) 123–126

3. Daniel, AE. *Preventing Suicide in Prison: A Collaborative Responsibility of Administrative, Custodial, and Clinical Staff.* Journal of American Academy of Psychiatry and the Law 34 [2] (2006) 165–175

4. Schaller, G, Zimmermann, C, and Raymond, L. *Risk factors in self-injurious behavior in a Swiss prison.* Sozialund Präventivmedizin 41(1996) 249–256

5. Kerkhof, AJ and Bernasco, W. *Suicidal Behavior in Jails and Prisons in The Netherlands: Incidence, Characteristics, and Prevention.* Suicide and Life-Threatening Behavior 20 (1990) 123–137

6. Perr, IN. *Suicide litigation and risk management.* Bulletin of the American Academy of Psychiatry and the Law 13 (1985) 209–19

7. Fruehwald, S, Eher, R, and Frottier P. *What Was the Relevance of Previous Suicidal Behavior in Prison Suicides?* Canadian Journal of Psychiatry 46 (8) (2001) 763

8. He, XY, Felthous, AR, Holzer, CE, Nathan, P and Veasey, S. *Factors in prison suicide: One year study in Texas.* Journal of Forensic Sciences 46 (2001) 896–901

9. White, TW, Schimmel, DJ and Frickey, R. *A Comprehensive Analysis of Suicide in Federal Prisons: A Fifteen-Year Review.* Journal of Correctional Health Care 9 (2002) 321–43

10. Marcus, P and Alcabes, P: *Characteristics of suicides by inmates in an urban jail.* Hospital and Community Psychiatry 44 (1993) 256–261

11. Du Rand, CJ, Burtka, GJ, Federman, EJ, Haycox, JA, et al. *A quarter century of suicide in a major urban jail: Implications for community psychiatry.* American Journal of Psychiatry 152 (1995) 1077–1080

12. Topp, DO. *Suicide in Prison.* British Journal of Psychiatry 134 (1979) 24–27

13. Fulwiler, C, Forbes, C, Santangelo, SL and Folstein, M. *Self-mutilation and suicide attempt: Distinguishing features in prisoners.* Journal of the American Academy of Psychiatry and the Law 25 (1997) 69–77

14. Liebling, A. *Suicides in young prisoners: A summary.* Death Studies 17 (1993) 381–409

15. Daniel, AE and Fleming, J. *Serious Suicide Attempts in Correctional System and Preventive Strategies,* Journal of Psychiatry and Law 33 (2005) 227–247

16. Marzano, L, Hawton, K, Rivlin A, et al. *Prevention of Suicidal Behavior in Prisons, An Overview of Initiatives Based on a Systematic Review of Research on Near-Lethal Suicide Attempts.* CRISIS 37 (5) (2016) 323–334

17. Konrad, N, Daigle, MS, Daniel, AE, Dear, G, Frottier, P, Hayes LM, Kerkhof A, Liebling, A, and Sarchiapone, M. *Preventing Suicide in Prisons. Part I recommendations from the International Association for Suicide Prevention Task Force on Suicide in Prisons.* CRISIS 28 (3) (2007) 113–121

18. Brown, GK, Henrique, GR, Sosdjan, D and Beck, AT. *Suicide intent and accurate expectations of lethality of suicide attempts.* Journal of Counseling and Clinical Psychology 72 (2004) 1170–1174

19. Gunnell, D, Bennewith, O, Hawton K, Simkin, S and Kapur, N. *Epidemiology and Prevention of Suicide by hanging, A systematic review.* International Journal of Epidemiology 34 (2) (2005) 433–442

20. Clement R, et al. *Mechanism of Death in Hanging: A historical Review of the Evolution of Pathophysiological Hypothesis.* Journal of Forensic Science 55 (5) (2010) 1268–1271

21. Schneidman, E. *A Psychologic Theory of Suicide.* Psychiatric Annals 6(11) (1976) 5–66

22. Joiner, TE Jr, Van Orden, K A, Witte, T K, and Rudd, MD. *The interpersonal theory of suicide: Guidance for working with suicidal clients.* American Psychological Association (2009). https://doi.org/10.1037

23. Taylor, S. *Power of Purpose*, Psychologytoday.com, Posted on July 21, 2013

24. Maier, SF and Seligman, M. *Learned Helplessness at Fifty: Insights from Neuroscience,* Psychological Review 123 (4) (2016) 349–367

25. Beck, AT, Brown, G, Berchick, RJ, et al. *Relationship between hopelessness and ultimate suicide: A replication with psychiatric outpatients.* American Journal of Psychiatry 147 (1990) 190–195

26. Erikson, EH. *Life Cycle Completed*, New York W.W. Norton & Company (1982)

27. Abramson, LY, Metalsky, GI and Alloy, LB. *Hopelessness depression: A theory-based subtype of depression.* Psychological Review 96(2) (1989) 358–372

28. Bonner, RL and Rich, AR. *Psychosocial vulnerability, life stress, and suicide ideation in a jail population: a cross-validation study.* Suicide Life Threatening Behavior 20 (3) (1990) 213–24

29. Gvion, Y and Apter, A. *Aggression, Impulsivity, and Suicide Behavior: A Review of the Literature.* Archives of Suicide Research 15(2) (2011) 93–112

30. Practice guideline for the assessment and treatment of patients with suicidal behaviors. American Journal of Psychiatry. 2003 Nov;160(11 Suppl):1-60.

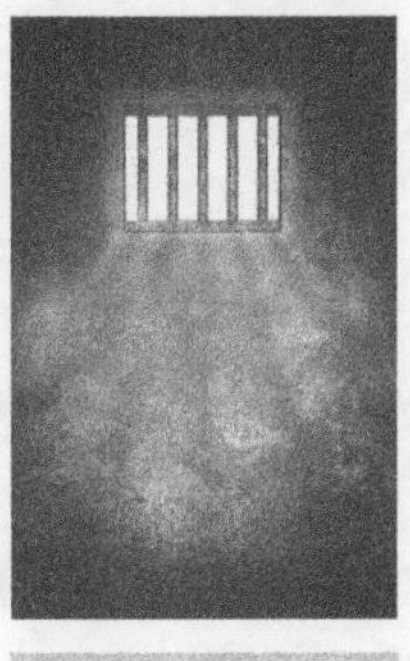

CHAPTER 2

SUICIDE: OVERVIEW AND PROBLEMS IN PREVENTION

The suicide of a few well-known and lesser-known inmates in American and Canadian correctional institutions during the last several years has attracted significant media and governmental scrutiny. These cases highlight the circumstances of suicide, failed assessment of risk factors, inadequate policies and procedures, and the lack of or difficulty in implementing prevention programs.

Aaron Hernandez, an NFL player, hanged himself in 2017 from a window in his cell in the Souza Baranowski Correctional Center, a maximum-security prison in Massachusetts approximately two days after his acquittal of a double homicide. He was already serving a life sentence. He left three notes before he died: one to his lawyer, one to his fiancé, and one to his daughter. A CT scan of his brain showed evidence of severe chronic traumatic encephalopathy (CTE). After his suicide, lawmakers raised questions about the increasing rate of suicide in Massachusetts prisons and the lack of access to mental health care for inmates in maximum-security cells.

Sandra Bland, a twenty-eight-year-old African American woman, died in the Waller County Jail in 2015 in Texas, three days after a trooper arrested her during a routine traffic stop. Although there were questions about the manner of her death, it was ruled a suicide by hanging. She had a history of a suicide attempt by overdose with pills and had a prior diagnosis of major depression. A handwritten jail screening form completed by an officer showed that she responded to a question on depression: "Are you feeling this way now?" Bland answered, "Yes." When asked whether she was considering suicide on the day of her arrest, she said, "No." The intake form showed that she was on levetiracetam (Keppra), an antiepileptic medication.

The *Washington Post*[1] reported that some of the documents from the jail appeared to contain contradictory information. Bland marked on the self-reported screening form that she had thoughts of killing herself the year before, and she was feeling very depressed on the day of her arrest. However, the computerized suicide assessment, completed by a correctional officer, listed "No" to questions on suicidal thoughts during the preceding year, depression in the past, and on the day of her arrest.

A "medical intake" form completed a few hours later, yet again showed a discrepancy in the information included in her self-report and the correctional officer's report. It listed "No" to the question about "attempted suicide." Ms. Bland's death triggered an investigation into the Waller County Jail practice, which showed non-compliance by jail officials with its policy regarding suicide training. Notably, the officers lacked the required two hours of suicide prevention training and inmate observation procedures.

"Craigslist Killer" Philip Haynes Markoff, a former second-year medical student, committed suicide in a Massachusetts jail in 2010 while awaiting trial. Before his death, he wrote three suicide notes: one on the day of his arrest; the second when his fiancé broke up with him; and the third when his wedding would have taken place. He used one of the jail's disposable razors to slash his wrists and a major artery in his leg. He wrapped the wound on his wrist in a garbage bag and tied another garbage bag tightly around his neck to suffocate himself. While in jail, he had been on suicide watch at various times.

In 2007, Ashley Smith, a nineteen-year-old teenager under suicide watch in a federal correctional institution in Canada, committed suicide by self-strangulation with a piece of cloth. In violation of the suicide protocol, she was not seen for forty-five minutes prior to the discovery of her death. Multiple investigations and reviews of care at the institution followed. The warden and assistant warden were fired. The Smith family filed a lawsuit against Canada's Correctional Service for negligence, which was settled out of court. Howard Sapers,[2] a correctional investigator, recommended provisions for mental health care to inmates, training for correctional officers, managing inmates' self-injurious behaviors, administrative segregation, mental health consultation, and the transfer of seriously mentally ill inmates to a specialized psychiatric unit.

Inmate suicides often cost correctional officers their jobs if an investigation confirms negligence or violation of standard practice. In 2015, five officers in the Licking County Jail in Newark, Ohio, lost their jobs after an inmate committed suicide and several other inmates attempted suicide. CBS-affiliate WBNS reported that the officers resigned after an investigation found that one officer had not checked the inmates as required and then falsified records.

The aforementioned cases illustrate the problems of delayed access to care, failure to identify suicide risk, lack of officer training, inaccurate documentation, and poor management of inmates' self-injurious behaviors.

Currently, no statewide organization exists to monitor jail policies and procedures. However, jails and statewide correctional systems may seek voluntary accreditation from National Commission on Correctional Health Care (NCCHC), a national organization that sets standards for best practice in jails and prisons. States including Texas, New York, and California have appointed commissions and inspectors to oversee their operations. Pennsylvania and Illinois prescribe jails must follow state suicide prevention policies. However, no guarantee exists those jails will follow the national or state guidelines.

After the Sandra Bland incident and a fifty-state survey of jail-suicide standards, Michele Deitch of the LBJ School of Public Affairs commented that "... formal and comprehensive external oversight—in the form of inspections and routine monitoring of conditions that affect the rights of prisoners—is truly rare in this country."[21]

After the fact, Texas enacted Texas Senate Bill 1849, known as the Sandra Bland Act, which requires that all deaths in jails be investigated by an independent law enforcement agency and, further, that inmates with mental health and substance abuse problems be diverted to mental health care and substance abuse treatment.

OVERVIEW

The increasing rate of custodial suicide has garnered a high degree of attention from researchers and policymakers. Several social, legal, policy, and programmatic events may explain the increasing interest. After the Community Mental Health Act of 1963, the resulting deinstitutionalization of the mentally ill led to a high criminal incarceration rate, even for minor offenses. Since the 1980s, jails and prisons have become de facto mental institutions. At the front end of the criminal justice system, lack of widespread use of diversion programs such as mental health and drug courts caused more people with psychiatric disorders to enter prisons. At the back end, almost 50% of released inmates "recycle" through the process every three years because of inadequate treatment and rehabilitation in the outside community.

Since late 1970s, several prisoner-initiated class-action lawsuits demanded access to reasonable medical and mental health care and rights and privileges. Prisoners are constitutionally mandated to receive reasonable and adequate medical and mental health care. Since 1976, landmark Supreme Court and federal court decisions have established necessary markers for proper medical and mental health care in the U.S. correctional system.

A court decision in 1980 by Judge William Wayne Justice in *Ruiz v. Estelle*[3] led the way, establishing suicide prevention programs in prisons. Justice found that the Texas prison system had "no program whatsoever for identification, treatment, or supervision of inmates with suicidal tendencies." This and other lawsuits led to screening programs for suicidal inmates. Yet the rate of suicide among inmates remains high compared with suicide rates in the outside community. The American Correctional Associations (ACA), American Psychiatric Association (APA), and the NCCHC have produced standards for medical and mental health care, support services, treatment paradigms, and designs for medical infirmaries in jails and prisons.

Inmates constitute a special "social" group due to their custody status, which obligates the state to protect them from harm. However, inmates assume some responsibility for accessing care. They are required to submit a Medical Services Request (MSR) form if they have concerns, symptoms, or merely want to visit with a medical or mental health provider. Inmates who are potentially imminently dangerous to themselves or others constitute an exception to the need for voluntary request.

The United States has the highest incarceration rate in the world
In the United States (as of March 2020), there were 1,833 state prisons, 110 federal prisons, 1,772 juvenile facilities, 3,134 local jails, 218 immigration detention facilities, 80 Indian Country jails, and a few military prisons.

The National Prisoner Statistics program (NPS) has collected an annual prisoner count since 1926. The total incarcerated population comprises all inmates in prisons, jails, and detention facilities. The Bureau of Justice Statistics (BJS) reported[4] that, in 2016, the total number people held in custody in the U.S. was 2,162,400, translating to an overall incarceration rate of 830 per 100,000 U.S. residents.

At midyear 2019, local jails in the U.S. held 734,500 inmates[5], down from a peak of 785,500 inmates in 2008. About 65% (480,700) of jail inmates were awaiting court action on a current charge, while the remaining 35% (253,700) were serving a sentence or awaiting sentencing on a conviction.

The jail incarceration rate decreased 13% from 2008 to 2019, declining from 258 to 224 inmates per 100,000 U.S. residents. Local jails reported 10.3 million admissions in 2019, which was 24% lower than the 13.6 million admissions in 2008. The total prison population in the U.S. declined from 1,464,400 at year-end 2018 to 1,430,800 at year-end 2019.[6] On average, the U.S. has approximately 2.2 million people in jails and prisons combined.

By comparison, the Council of Europe Annual Penal Statistics report from 2013 shows the median prison population across Europe was 133 per 100,000; 188 in Canada; 130 in Australia; 190 in New Zealand; and 51 in Japan.

It is striking that, while just 4.4% of the world population lives in the U.S., it has 22% of all prisoners in the world. However, as noted above, the incarceration rate in the U.S. may be declining due to recent reforms. The incarceration rate calculated as the number of inmates per 100,000 people in the United States in 2016 was 830, a decline from 860 in 2009.

About 16% to 20% of the inmate population is seriously mentally ill, diagnosed with schizophrenia, bipolar disorder, schizoaffective disorder, major depressive disorder, and other psychotic disorders. With more mentally ill in jails and prisons, more suicides occur.

SUICIDE RATE

World Health Organization (WHO) statistics show that approximately 800,000 people who are not incarcerated die by suicide worldwide every year. In the U.S., 42,773 people died from suicide in 2014, compared with 29,199 in 1999.[7] In 2020, 45,173 died by suicide, making it the tenth leading cause of death by people of all ages. It is the second leading cause of death among people between 15 and 29 years old. However, White men over 55 are at the highest risk of dying by suicide.

The suicide rate in jails and prisons is usually compared with the commonly accepted national general population rate of 12 per 100,000; however, the comparison is inaccurate because of the disparity in the distribution of men and women in jails and prisons. When this general population rate of 12 per 100,000 is broken down by gender, the rate for men is 18 and for women is 6. Therefore, the correctional rate of 18 to 20 is comparable with the rate among men in the general population.[8]

The suicide rate in correctional facilities is usually calculated by the number of suicides by the average daily population (ADP) extrapolated to 100,000. ADP is determined on the daily count at a specified time of the day, often midnight, when the daily count is taken. The ADP-based calculation has recently been questioned as to whether it is the best way to calculate the rate: This method often does not consider the total at-risk population, which includes those who spend a few hours in jail or lock up and are released on bond.

Underreporting of suicide may, of course, underestimate the suicide rate. If a suicide victim is found and rushed to the hospital, only to die there, records may not show that the victim committed suicide in jail or prison. Also, some facilities choose not to report some deaths that can be linked to failures in the intake process (e.g., deaths related to drugs and alcohol). Bureau of Justice statistics show that, in recent years, jails have had increased rates of "drug or alcohol intoxication deaths." In

2012, there were fifty-seven drug- and alcohol-related deaths. In 2013, there were seventy.

For several decades before 2000, the U.S. prison suicide rate ranged from 18 to 40 per 100,000. This rate has declined considerably since 2001. The annual average rate of suicides from 2001 to 2016 was 17 deaths per 100,000 for male state prisoners and 13 deaths per 100,000 for female state prisoners.

Before 2000, the federal prisons had 10 to 17 suicides per 100,000.[9] Currently, the federal prisons have the lowest rate, with 10 per 100,000. The highest suicide rate is noted among death row inmates, with 146.5 per 100,000.[10]

The latest available statistics show a slightly improved rate in jails. The suicide rate declined from 52 to 46 deaths per 100,000 jail inmates.[11] In local jails overall, suicides make up 31% of all deaths. However, deaths due to suicide decreased 10% from 2015 to 2016. In 2016, as in prior years, 80% of jails reported no suicides, while 13% reported one, and 7% reported two or more. [11] In 2016, the number of deaths in jails by any cause was 1,071, a 1.9% decrease from the 1,092 deaths reported in 2015[11], with suicide at 332. Although there was a slight decrease in the number of suicides in jails, suicide was the leading cause of death in local jails in 2016. Heart disease, however, was the second highest.[11]

In 2016, in state and federal prisons combined, the total number of deaths by any cause, was 4,117.[12] The number of deaths in state prisons rose 1.3% from 2015 to 2016 (from 3,682 to 3,729), while the number of deaths in federal prisons fell 15% (from 455 to 388). This marked the first decrease in deaths in federal prisons since 2012.

Each year from 2001 to 2016, an average of 88% of deaths in state prisons were due to natural causes, ranging from 89%

in 2001 to 86% in 2016. Over the same time span, an average of 11% of deaths in state prisons were due to unnatural causes (suicide, drug, or alcohol intoxication). Upon further research, this seems to be the case, as state prisons had 3,300 deaths by suicide from 2001–2016 while federal prisons had only 260.

The suicide rate in corrections has remained high, per the latest statistics in 2016, with the rate in jails at 46/100,000, in state prisons at 17/100,000, and federal prisons at 10 per 100,000. Except for the federal prisons, the rates remain high compared to the U.S. general population, making the incarcerated population a high-risk group for suicide. The latest report from Bureau of Justice, shows an uptick in suicide rate in jails and prisons as of 2019. The state and federal prisons showed a significant increase during the period between 2015 and 2019. The jail rate showed no increase during the same period, though the overall rate increased by 13% between 2001 and 2019. Still, inmates in jails and prisons remain a high risk group for suicide.[22][1]

---

1 From 2001 to 2019, the number of suicides increased 85% in state prisons, 61% in federal prisons, and 13% in local jails. During 2010–19, suffocation, including hanging and self-strangulation, accounted for nearly 90% of suicide deaths in local jails. During 2015–19, about 12% of deaths by suicide in local jails occurred within the first 24 hours of incarceration, a decrease from almost 22% during 2000–04. The average suicide rate for white inmates in local jails was 93 per 100,000 during the 5-year period of 2015–19, which is 5 times the rate for black inmates (18 per 100,000) and more than 3 times the rate for Hispanic inmates (26 per 100,000). Almost 60% of state prisoners who died by suicide during 2001–19 were white. During 2001–19, state prisoners who had been sentenced for a violent offense accounted for almost 72% of suicides in state prisons. During 2015–19, about 75% of suicides in state prisons and 64% of suicides in federal prisons occurred after the first year of imprisonment. Persons serving time in federal prison for weapons offenses and sex offenses each accounted for about 20% of suicides in federal facilities during 2015–19.

COMMON PROBLEMS IN SUICIDE PREVENTION

The responsibility for suicide prevention has traditionally been placed squarely on mental health staff. Experience has shown that in the absence of administrative support and involvement, their efforts may be doomed to fail. Correctional employees, including mental health staff and correctional officers, have joint responsibility for ensuring inmates' health and safety, and they are increasingly held liable, individually and collectively, when they fail in their duty.

The commonly identified problems in suicide prevention include the following.

1. *Misidentification of at-risk inmates*

   Misidentification of the potential at-risk population at every point in the process of incarceration from arrest through release is a significant issue. Most clinicians and officers are naturally perceptive and empathetic and can spot suicidal inmates. Occasionally, they ignore their "third sense" through neglect-fulness or by intentionally, rationalizing: "Why do I save these guys who caused so much pain to their victims?" or "They are the scum of society; if they want to kill themselves, let them do it." or "Why should the state spend so much money to take care of them?" A correctional officer who believes that all prisoners, regardless of mental illness, are manipulative, attention-seeking, and antisocial may miss an opportunity to intervene in crises and prevent an inmate from committing suicide.[13]

2. *Lack of standard screening instrument*

   A lack of a standardized suicide screening questionnaire may result in inadequate risk assessment. When there is a questionnaire, screeners often spend insufficient time completing it. Mass screenings are often conducted in a hurried fashion in busy jails with numerous detainees awaiting processing. Failure to explore key items in the questionnaire regarding current suicidal ideation, past suicide attempts, medication history, and date of last use of drugs, particularly opiates, may negatively impact detainees' care. More important, inadequate screenings may result in not placing a genuinely suicidal detainee/inmate on suicide watch.

3. *Inadequate mental health assessment and treatment planning*
A major finding in the history of many inmates who commit suicide is a lack of or inadequate mental health assessment and treatment planning. Although many facilities mandate development of treatment plans, a lack of consistent implementation of a treatment planning directive delays appropriate care.

A proper mental health assessment consisting of a detailed mental status examination and diagnosis consistent with DSM-5 and carried out by a qualified mental health professional supports proper treatment planning of potentially suicidal inmates. Treatment planning consistent with standard of care provides directions regarding medication management, level of supervision, watch, and therapy needs.

4. *Inadequate and or lack of periodic suicide risk assessment*
Often, suicide risk assessment in jails and prisons consists of limited queries regarding an inmate's suicidal thoughts and plans—instead of a detailed examination of all risk factors in order to arrive at a reasoned conclusion of whether

an inmate presents a suicide risk. Lack of risk assessment at certain focal points, such as a transfer from another facility, court proceedings, new charges, sentencing, and external psychosocial stressors, may result in failure to identify inmates whose risk might be in response to changing circumstances and events.

5. ***Discontinuation of psychotropic medication at entry to jail or prison***

   Many inmates enter a jail or prison on prescription medications. These may include psychotropic agents and life-sustaining medications such as antihypertensives, antidiabetics, angina medications, and breathalyzers. On occasion, psychotropics are discontinued abruptly, causing severe withdrawal symptoms, including increasing anxiety and agitation, thus predisposing the inmate to suicidal behaviors. Abrupt discontinuation of psychotropic medication was cited in a successful deliberate indifference lawsuit.[14]

6. ***Failure to obtain medical and psychiatric records from community sources***

   The failure to obtain records from community sources may cause a delay in care and adversely affect determination of supervision, watch requirements, and proper treatment planning. Prior psychiatric and medical records provide critical information regarding the inmates' past psychiatric history, prior suicide attempts, treatment received, and medications. The most critical information includes past suicide attempt history, recent hospitalizations (including any involuntary commitment), substance withdrawal, and medications.

7. *Failure to provide "bridge medications"*

Understandably, it takes time to obtain an inmate's past psychiatric records or verify medications. However, based on the history provided by the inmate and clinical information obtained by a nurse or screener, it is appropriate to prescribe psychotropic medications to "bridge" the period until the required information becomes available. Failure to provide bridge medication may delay inmate health care. Sometimes it leads to precipitation of withdrawal symptoms or recurrence of psychiatric symptoms, including suicidal thoughts.

8. *Delay in psychiatric care*

Delayed psychiatric care can be described as an intentional disregard of an inmate's serious medical need. Various correctional standards emphasize the importance of critical time frames in screening, referral, and evaluation. Intake is conducted the day of a detainee's arrival at a jail or prison. Suicide screening takes place in the first twenty-four hours. A mental health evaluation is completed within twenty-four hours of referral from the screener. A psychiatric evaluation is done within fourteen days, except on emergency referrals. Medical Services Requests (MSR) are responded to within three business days, except in emergencies. Follow-up psychiatric contact is generally completed within thirty days. Delay in these time frames may lead to poor care and potential suicidal behaviors.

Delay in responding to a Medical Response Request is yet another situation that may be associated with suicidal thoughts and an inmate feeling "nobody cares."

9. *Failure to implement detoxification protocol*

Often, arrestees enter a jail intoxicated with alcohol or under the influence of opiates—including heroin, and meth-amphetamine or a combination of substances. Recognizing a state of intoxication and initiating detoxification proto-col prevents distressing withdrawal symptoms, which predisposes inmates to suicidal ideation and behaviors. Sometimes, a state of intoxication may be identified, but pro-viders may fail to place the detainee in medically supported withdrawal protocol.[15]

10. *Falsification of suicide watch logs*

A more common problem is the falsification of suicide watch logs. Logs must be completed every 15 minutes or less, at staggered intervals. It is common to find inaccurately recorded suicide watch logs. For example, a log may reflect log entries exactly at the prescribed 15 minute intervals. The defense loses many lawsuits due to falsified documentation of suicide watch logs.

11. *Failure of communication*

Failure of communication is a key issue in suicide preven-tion. This may occur at many levels: between the arresting officer and the booking officer; the booking officer and the mental health screener; the nursing staff and the psychiatrist; and the scheduler of appointments and the psychiatrist. Failure to schedule a potentially suicidal inmate with the psychiatrist may delay a critical psychiatric evaluation, risk assessment, and intervention.

An arresting officer may have a prima facie or visceral impression that an arrestee is suicidal. Unless the officer communicates his or her impression to the booking officer, this valuable information is missed. Some suicide screening questionnaires include a question to summarize the arresting officer's impression.

Today, screening questionnaires are computerized. Should a suicide alert be posted on the computer by a screener, if there is no mechanism in the computer to display the alert, at the time of evaluation, the mental health professional would be unaware of the alerts. Rarely, miscommunication may occur in the transfer of medication orders to the Medication Administration Record.

Occasionally, a spouse or significant other may call a jail or prison to communicate a concern about the next of kin's potential suicide risk. Such calls are to be documented and the information given to the mental health providers for further action. If the jails or prisons have no system to document such calls, information crucial for suicide prevention may be lost.

Daniel and Fleming reported that 60% of inmates communicated their intent to outside people, but those who received the information often failed to communicate to the jail because they did not take it seriously, creating yet another communication problem.[16]

Compartmentalization of documentation by the medical and mental health staff and that of the custody staff is the norm in jails and prisons. This restricts sharing critical information between the officers and mental health providers. Health Insurance Portability and Accountability Act (HIPAA) regulations may preclude sharing of protected information. However, if knowledge of an inmate's mental health conditions and prior suicidal behavior is kept from the officers, they have no meaningful way to work with the inmate at risk. Often, after a tragic event, the correctional officers regret their perceived neglect. Most officers acknowledge that suicide prevention is "everybody's responsibility; we are in it together."

A different level of communication problem may occur between inmates and officers. Some inmates in distress may try to reach an officer via intercom in their cell. Failure to respond to the intercom contact may convince the inmate that "nobody cares." I know of a situation where an inmate tried to reach the control room via the intercom, which was ignored. In another situation, the intercom call display in the control room was muted. In both situations, the inmates killed themselves a few minutes after their attempts to contact the officers were thwarted.

Systematic communication among stakeholders can save lives. Reasonable communication between mental health and correctional staff is desirable. The intercom system must be functional.

12. *Classification Issues*

Typically, in a department of corrections, prisons are classified as minimum, medium, and maximum security, and inmates are assigned to the facilities that provide the level of security and custody an inmate requires. Jail inmates are classified as low, medium, and high custody risk, based on the type of crime, and tendency for elopement, violence, and security disturbance. While inmates with mental illness may be considered to have special needs, mental illness is usually not a major consideration in custody risk assignment.

Classification of inmates, assignment of institutions (prisons), cell selection, cell movement, and placement in disciplinary segregation is entirely assigned to the correctional staff. The mental health staff usually provides input to the classification staff in assigning mentally ill inmates. From a suicide prevention standpoint, such arrangements cause significant challenges, particularly when interdisciplinary communication is lacking. Failure to accept or provide mental health input may impact cell assignment of a potentially suicidal inmate. Correctional officers primarily conduct inmate classification and cell assignment.

13. *Lack of implementation of policy and procedures*

Besides training, lack of implementation of facility policies and procedures, particularly those related to suicide prevention, are the most significant issue in suicide prevention.[17]

14. *Training*

Proper training of correctional officers and mental health staff in identifying the inmate at-risk is the single most significant factor in preventing suicide.

In almost every lawsuit involving suicide, the lack of training of officers and mental health staff is cited to support a deliberate indifference or medical negligence claim. The claims may link the staff's lack of or poor training on risk factors, their lack of knowledge of suicide prevention policies and procedures, and their failure to implement these policies and procedures to the inmate's suicide. Such an argument may be strong in cases where a cluster of suicides occur during a period in the same jail where a recent claimant died. Sometimes, the lawsuit may claim the suicide rate in a particular jail or prison exceeds that of similar institutions during the same period. Cluster suicide may reflect the staff's lack of training.

SYSTEM ISSUES IN SUICIDE PREVENTION

The increasing prevalence of seriously mentally ill inmates in the context of inadequate resources and staffing creates major treatment challenges for health-care providers who must ensure that their mission is carried out without compromising their professional standards.

1. *Access to care*

Suicide prevention efforts may be hampered by limited access to mental health care and treatment opportunities. Some large jails and most prisons have a designated psychiatric stabilization unit where a suicidal inmate can be provided with crisis intervention and medication adjustment. In such units, mental health staff perform suicide risk assessment, provide supportive therapy, and allow the inmate to vent his or her frustration. Traditional psychotherapy can be extremely helpful for inmates but may not be possible due to limited staffing and budgetary constraints.

Some severely disturbed inmates may be transferred to a local state mental hospital, though the recent trend is to provide mental health treatment in the jail or prison. To that extent, creating an acute care psychiatric unit in the facility may enhance implementation of psychiatric treatment. Some grossly psychotic and non-compliant patients who are dangerous to themselves or others may benefit from involuntary medication treatment consistent with the *Washington v. Harper* criteria.[18]

2. *Privatization*

Beginning in the late 1990s, privatization of mental health and medical services at jails and prisons has gained strength. The reasons for this trend include escalating health-care costs and staff expense, lack of available qualified correctional health care professionals, lack of visionary correctional leadership (with exceptions) in government-run jails and prisons, and mental-health-services-related litigation.

3. *Access to medication*

Inmate access to effective psychiatric medications is critical for suicide prevention. Medications are the treatment mainstay of mentally ill inmates. Most psychiatrists choose antidepressants, antipsychotics, antianxiety medications, and sleep promoting agents and medications for side effects that are consistent with community treatment standards. Due to abusive potential, benzodiazepines are not generally prescribed in jails and prisons.

Pharmaceutical costs increase 15–20% annually. Some private contractors target prescription drugs to cut costs aggressively via a restricted formulary. Some insist the psychiatrists prescribe less expensive older generation antipsychotics and antidepressants rather than expensive, albeit effective, newer medications. Cost-containment measures are mediated via a concurrent nonformulary review process, placing undue burden on psychiatrists.

Newer medications improve inmates' quality of life. More important, they help reduce overall health-care costs by reducing long-term hospitalization, emergency admissions to psychiatric units, and indirect costs associated with inmate transportation to psychiatric facilities.

Contractors' profit motives may trump quality and thus compromise ethical standards and practice in jails and prisons. Some contractors keep key staff positions unfilled, potentially jeopardizing patient care and suicide prevention efforts.

The preferred method for cost stabilization and containment must include the establishment of diagnostic and treatment parameters for mental disorders consistent with American Psychiatric Association recommendations. Other measures must include stringent peer review and proper quality-assurance activities, including monitoring long- and short-term side effects.[19]

4. *Substance abuse treatment*

Systematic substance abuse treatment and rehabilitation, which is a significant suicide prevention effort, is sorely lacking in jails and prisons. Medication Assisted Treatment (MAT) with naltrexone and similar anti-craving agents for alcohol dependence, and buprenorphine/naloxone (Suboxone) for opiate dependence may enhance the potential for successful reentry of many inmates into the outside community and decrease recidivism. Only a small fraction of inmates in the correctional system receive medication assisted treatment.

Inmates arrested for drug- or alcohol-related charges experience a reprieve when the access to the offending substance is cut off. Over several days or weeks during detention, the withdrawal symptoms dissipate and the inmate regains a semblance of normalcy. However, the cessation of craving is only temporary.

The first month after their release from prison, inmates are increasingly vulnerable to substance abuse relapse as they enter a cue-rich environment of drugs and alcohol. Some newly released inmates are particularly vulnerable to suicide immediately after release. American psychiatrist and neurologist Abraham Wikler (1910–1981)[20] eloquently pointed out the occurrence of physical symptoms akin to acute withdrawal, known as conditioned abstinence, when the inmates return to their familiar environment, triggering relapse. The newly released inmate has a twelve-fold risk of overdosing and dying within the first thirty days of release. This is especially true with opioid-use disorders. Incarcerated subjects gradually lose their tolerance to the opioids. If they go back to using the same dose of opioids as at the time of arrest, there is a high risk of overdose death.

Addictive disorders get embedded in the memory, emotional, and motivational circuits of the "pleasure," or limbic system. The addiction gets "hard-wired" and can powerfully reemerge in response to cues and triggers any time after remission, for example, when an inmate is released from incarceration. When a subject is incarcerated, the addiction goes into an "incubator." Each time the patient thinks, talks, dreams, or fantasizes about drug or alcohol use, he/she triggers cravings and feeds the addiction "hiding" in the incubator. The cravings become stronger and more frequent as the inmate is close to being released. It is a well-known fact: the priorities upon release are food, sex, drugs, or alcohol. We have often heard this phenomenon aptly described as: You are in jail or prison, but your addiction is in the parking lot doing push-ups and getting stronger!

Given this background, there is a compelling reason to provide evidence-based treatment almost immediately upon incarceration. Effective withdrawal management followed by the appropriate anti-craving medications, such as buprenorphine or naltrexone, will break the cycle of passively feeding the addictive disorder. This will allow inmates to be more actively involved in behavioral therapies designed to prevent relapse when released. It is critical for inmates with substance abuse disorders to receive the appropriate anti-craving medications and referral to treatment centers upon release to continue treatment in a seamless manner. This is consistent with the long-standing policy of giving inmates appropriate antipsychotic medications upon release. This cost-effective approach has several benefits, including the reduced risk of suicides, drug overdoses, violence, and a lower incidence of recidivism.

ROLE OF MENTAL HEALTH STAFF

The onus of suicide prevention in jails and prisons falls on the mental health and medical staff. Most facilities employ an organized medical staff with a medical director and a health services administrator (HSA) to oversee inmates' medical care. The medical director may be a direct employee of the jail or an outside contractor. The mental health staff is organized under a mental health director, a social worker, or a psychologist. A mental health unit director oversees and manages the mental health services in each facility. The unit mental health director collaborates with the HSA. He or she must work with the correctional officers in suicide prevention efforts.

In most jails and prisons, medical and mental health services are privatized. For some jails, private mental health agencies supply the entire mental health staff. About twenty-five states and several large urban jails contract with private vendors for correctional health-care services. Currently, Texas use medical schools exclusively. Georgia uses medical schools for medical care and contracts with a private mental health vendor. New Jersey contracts with a medical school for mental health and with a large private vendor for medical care. Contractors in other states range from small private vendors for mental health services with various agreements for staffing and services to large private correctional health-care companies providing both medical and mental health care.

Although the policies and procedures pertaining to mental health care and suicide prevention may be developed by the vendor, they should be approved and implemented according to a contract between each facility and the vendor. The contract between the Department of Corrections and large private vendors specifies the operating procedures, organization of mental health and medical units, quality improvement procedures, service audits, and the required staffing in each of the correctional centers under the state's governance. The contract also specifies the mental health staff's qualifications and credentials, including those of the director of mental health, psychiatrists, psychologists, "qualified mental health professionals," nurses, and various paraprofessionals, consistent with individual state's administrative codes and statutes. The state approves the pharmacy, the formulary, and the medication approval procedures for individual inmates. Policies and procedures regarding suicide prevention, access to mental health care, medication administration, emergency crisis management, and mortality and morbidity reviews are developed and approved by the contractor and the vendor. In addition, the state supervises and audits the entire operation, so the contractor follows and abides by the contract's specifications for the provision of quality services to inmates.

Psychiatrists play a unique role in suicide prevention
Depending on a jail's size, psychiatrists may be hired on a part-time or full-time basis. Large jails may employ several full-time psychiatrists. Psychiatrists play a unique role in suicide prevention by providing psychiatric evaluation, suicide risk identification and assessment, medication management, and crisis management. Prior to an initial psychiatric evaluation, the nursing staff obtains the inmate's past and current medication history and verifies those histories with the community psychiatric provider. Sometimes, they contact pharmacies to verify medications. The inmate signs a Release of Information (ROI) form to obtain his or her medical and mental health records.

With input from the mental health team, a nurse or a scheduler develops a daily list of inmates to be seen by the psychiatrist. Each day's list may include inmates in crisis and those considered acutely dangerous to themselves or others. At every diagnostic or therapeutic encounter, the psychiatrist, psychologist, and social worker must assess each inmate's suicide risk. All mental health providers are required to promptly document every inmate contact. Psychologists and social workers evaluate segregated inmates for suitability to continue such confinement. Continued solitary confinement is highly stressful and may precipitate acute mental symptoms in some inmates.

CONCLUSION

Suicide prevention efforts in jails and prisons are complex processes involving individual professionals' specific responsibilities. Addressing system issues by developing and administering treatment programs for mentally and substance-abusing suicidal inmates is equally important.

REFERENCES

1. *Washington Post*, Morning Mix, July 23, 2015, by Elahe Izadi and Abby Phillip "Sandra Bland Previously Attempted Suicide, Jail Documents Say"
2. Sapers, H. *A Preventable Death*. Report of the Office of the Correctional Investigator, Ottawa (2008)
3. Ruiz v. Estelle, 503 F. Supp. 1265 (S.D. Tex. 1980)
4. Assessing Inmate Cause of Death: Deaths in Custody Reporting Program and National Death Index (ojp.gov) (2016)
5. https://www.bjs.gov/index.cfm?ty=pbdetail&iid=7267
6. https://www.bjs.gov/content/pub/pdf/p19.pdf
7. https://www.cdc.gov.nchs/products/databriefs/db241.htm
8. Daniel, AE. *Preventing suicide in prison: a collaborative responsibility of administrative, custodial, and clinical*

staff. Journal of the American Academy of Psychiatry and Law 34(2) (2006) 165–175

9. White, TW, Schimmel, DJ, Frickey, R. *A Comprehensive Analysis of Suicide in Federal Prisons: A Fifteen-Year Review.* Journal of Correctional Health Care 9 (2002) 321–45

10. Lester, D, Danto, BL: *Suicide Behind Bars: Prediction and Prevention. Philadelphia: The Charles Press* (1993) 18–21

11. https://www.bjs.gov/content/pub/pdf/mlj0016st.pdf

12. https://www.bjs.gov.content/pub/pdf.msfp0116st.pdf

13. Daniel, AE. *Commentary: Decision-making by front-line service providers—attitudinal or contextual.* Journal of American Academy of Psychiatry and Law 32(4) (2004) 386–9

14. Steele v. Shah, 87 F.3d 1266 (11th Cir. 1996)

15. Estate of Kempf v. Washington City, No. CV.15-1125, 2018, WL4354547

16. Daniel, AE and Fleming J. *Serious Suicide Attempts in Correctional System and Preventive Strategies,* Journal of Psychiatry and Law, 33 (2005)227–247

17. Woodward v. Myres, No. 00 C 6010, 99 C 0290 (N.D. Ill. Dec. 4, 2002)

18. Washington v. Harper, 494 U.S. 210 (1990)

19. Daniel, AE. *Care of the mentally ill in prisons: Challenges and solutions, Editorial (invited).* Journal of American Academy of Psychiatry and Law 35(5) (2007) 406–409

20. Wikler, A. *Dynamics of drug dependence. Implications of conditioning theory for research and treatment.* Archives of General Psychiatry 28 (1973) 611–16

21. Michele Deitch, "But Who Oversees the Overseers?: The Status of Prison and Jail Oversight in the United States," American Journal of Criminal Law 207 (2020), p. 241.

22. Suicide in Local Jails and State and Federal Prisons, 2000–2019—Statistical Tables by Ann Carson, PhD. Bureau of Justice Statistics, https://bjs.ojp.gov/library /publications/list?series_filter=Mortality%20in%20 Local%20Jails%20and%20State%20Prisons

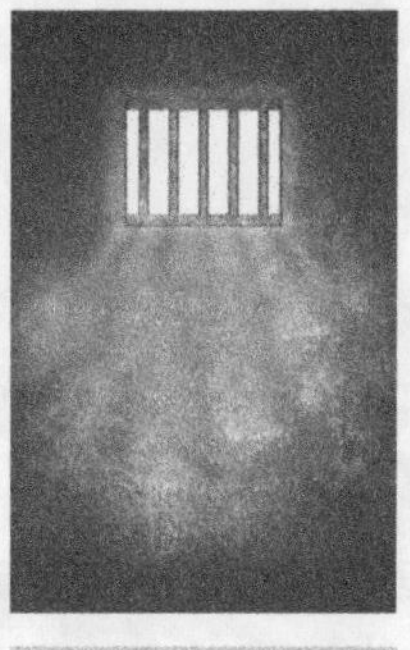

CHAPTER 3

BEST PRACTICES OF SUICIDE RISK ASSESSMENT

The U.S. Supreme Court, in *Estelle v. Gamble* in 1976,[1] paved the way for a prison to have a system of screening and evaluation in place for those in need of mental health treatment. Since then, the essential components of mental health screening and evaluation were set by the standards identified by the American Psychiatric Association (APA) and the National Commission on Correctional Health Care (NCCHC).

Upon admission to a jail or prison, all individuals should be given a screening for mental illness using a standard set of questions performed by a mental health professional or a trained correctional officer.

If screening reveals problems related to mental health, substance abuse, or suicidal ideation in an inmate, a mental health evaluation must occur.[2]

A MENTAL HEALTH EVALUATION SHOULD INCLUDE:

1. psychiatric history, including hospitalization and out-patient treatment;
2. current use of psychotropic medications, if any;
3. current suicidal ideation;
4. current and prior use of drugs and alcohol;
5. history of sex offenses;
6. history of violent behavior;
7. history of being victimized by violent behaviors;
8. history of special education placement;
9. history of seizures or head trauma;
10. emotional response to incarceration; and
11. intelligence testing for mental retardation.

This evaluation must occur within fourteen days and be conducted by a qualified mental health professional—a psychiatrist, psychologist, social worker, nurse, physician assistant, and any others permitted by law. While a trained correctional officer can perform the initial screening, a qualified mental professional must perform the mental health evaluation. The nature of the mental health professionals' credentials and their practice scope is defined in state statutes and administrative codes for mental health services.

Suicide risk assessment is a critical component of a comprehensive suicide prevention program in jails and prisons.[3, 4] While the program aims to screen, identify, assess, and monitor an inmate at potential risk, in practice, it is often limited to a screening questionnaire and brief inquiry of suicidal ideation at the time of clinical contact.

Most jail and prison clinical administrators recognize the importance of screening for inmate suicide risk. However, problems abound in selecting the appropriate screening instruments. Often, items that correlate with risk are not prioritized.

The process of suicide risk assessment in jails and prisons involves a clinician who identifies an inmate's risk and protective factors to modify them with treatment or programmatic interventions to manage the at-risk inmate.

Although clinicians are tasked with determining if an inmate will commit suicide, such prediction is not possible. The process requires the best possible methods and tools to identify at-risk inmates and intervene early. Screening instruments, even if used meticulously, yield high false positives. The positive predictive value of a suicide risk model in a large outpatient clinical setting is just 6%[5], which means seventeen individuals must receive intervention in order to save one life. This is cost-intensive.

No suicide prediction model exists in the correctional practice. Predicting suicide risk in jails and prisons relies on a clinically relevant assessment and management model—because the suicide of an inmate depends on situations and circumstances that are likely to change over time.

The purpose of suicide risk assessment is threefold:

1. Clinical
2. Meeting the standard of care
3. Determination of suicide vulnerability

Clinical:
An inmate's risk is assessed dimensionally, as low, moderate, and high, facilitating intervention to place the inmate

under suicide watch and instituting steps to mitigate the risk of suicide.

Standard of Care:

The standard of care on suicide risk assessment involves the correctional clinician. It falls into two broad categories[6]: professional and legal. Best practices and evidence-based assessment determine the professional standard of care consistent with the community and professional organizations' standards, including the American Psychiatric Association, American Correctional Association (ACA), and Joint Commission. An assessment that a clinician deviated from the standard of care is based on whether the clinician adhered to the best practice in performing the risk assessment. The legal standard involves whether the clinician took prudent and reasonable care in assessing the risk, as would a similarly trained individual under similar circumstances.

Suicide Vulnerability:

Various courts give great weight to the identification of factors that form the basis of a legal determination of suicide vulnerability of an inmate and to ultimately determine whether officers and clinicians ignored an inmate's vulnerability.[7, 8]

RISK FACTORS

The best practice-based suicide risk assessment relies on identifying an inmate's risk factors. In the community, high-risk groups for suicide include persons with psychiatric disorders and substance abuse, those newly diagnosed with serious physical illness, and those with previous suicide attempts. Detainees and prisoners represent a high-risk group.[9, 10]

Risk factors in jails and prisons differ from risk factors in the outside community in many ways. The principal predictors of inmate suicide include men (over age fifty-five), with previous near-lethal suicide attempts, alcohol and opioid withdrawal, intractable pain, depressive disorders with hopelessness, planning suicide attempt, high suicide intent, and ongoing psychiatric treatment. However, clinical experience, case reports, and retrospective studies[11] show an exhaustive list of risk factors affecting inmates. In settings where limited budgetary and staffing resources determine the level of services, a reliable screening instrument must be developed that meets the standard of care.

Inmate suicide risk factors can be divided into 1) Static (non-variable) factors; and 2) Dynamic (modifiable) factors. Dynamic factors act as immediate precipitants to suicide. Some factors are unique to jail inmates and some to prison inmates, as noted below.

A. *Static Risk Factors in Jails and Prisons*

1. Past suicide attempt(s)
2. A history of mental disorder
   a. Depressive disorder
   b. Bipolar disorder
   c. Anxiety disorder
   d. Schizophrenia and other psychotic disorders
3. Post-Traumatic Stress Disorder (PTSD)
4. Traumatic Brain Injury (TBI)
5. History of inpatient psychiatric treatment
6. Current psychiatric medication use
7. Diagnosis of substance abuse

      a. Alcohol abuse

      b. Heroin/opiate abuse

      c. Methamphetamine use

8. Chronic medical condition

      a. HIV/AIDS

      b. Intractable pain

9. Family history of suicide

      a. Suicide in first-degree relatives

10. High profile in society

      a. Loss of status

11. First arrest/first prison time

12. History of child abuse

      a. Physical abuse

      b. Sexual abuse

13. History of suicidal thoughts

14. History of violent behavior

15. Sex offender status

16. Homicidal ideation

17. Requested protective status

18. Victim of sexual assault

19. Lack of family connection

20. Unemployment

21. Poverty

B. *Dynamic (modifiable) Factors*

1. Agitation

2. Acute anxiety

3. Current pain

4. Current suicidal ideation

5. Current suicidal plan
6. Fear of own safety
7. Hopelessness
8. Overwhelming guilt
9. Helplessness
10. Feeling trapped
11. Feeling like a burden
12. Lack of compliance with treatment
13. Problem-solving deficit
14. Recent loss of a loved one
15. Sleep problems
16. Social isolation
17. Change in appetite
18. Impulsivity
19. Sudden change in mental status
20. Giving away possessions
21. New charges and the prospect of lengthy incarceration

C. *Factors Specific to Jails*

1. Alcohol intoxication and withdrawal
2. Opiate intoxication and withdrawal
3. Benzodiazepine intoxication and withdrawal
4. First arrest and loss of status in society
5. Solitary confinement
6. Loss of family connectedness
7. Impending divorce
8. Loss of custody of children
9. Added charges and the prospect of a lengthy sentence and transfer to prison

10. Denial of bond or high bond

D. *Factors specific to prisons*

1. Placement in maximum security
2. Change of custody status from low to high
3. Solitary confinement
4. Victim of prison rape
5. Additional charges and the prospect of a lengthy sentence

DEMOGRAPHIC VARIABLES

More incarcerated men than women die by suicide—although more women attempt suicide. Incarcerated women tend to have a higher rate of mental illness. Therefore, mentally ill female inmates have a higher rate of completed suicide compared with women with no mental illness.[9] Suicide prevention efforts should focus on women with a history of suicidal behavior, emotional problems, and diagnosed psychiatric illness.

The relationship of race to suicide is undetermined, although more incarcerated Whites die by suicide than do any other race. The disparity appears to be significant, considering the disproportionate number of Blacks in jails and prisons.

TYPE OF FACILITY

There are over five thousand jails and prisons in the United States, with a wide range of inmate capacity. Suicide occurs in small jails, lockups, large jails, state prisons, and federal prisons. However, prisoners in jails and smaller prisons may have increased risk of suicide. In 2015,[12] the suicide rate in the county jail population in the U.S. was 47/100,000. The nation's smallest jails have a suicide rate greater than six times that of the nation's largest jails.[13]

Maximum security prisons have a higher rate of suicide compared with medium- and minimum-security prisons.[14]

PRETRIAL DETAINEES VS. SENTENCED PRISONERS

Pretrial detainees have a higher suicide rate compared with sentenced prisoners. They are typically male, young, unmarried, and usually arrested for substance-related offenses. They are generally intoxicated at the time of arrest and commit suicide within a few hours of detention. The most cited reasons for the higher rate among detainees include sudden isolation, the shock of imprisonment, lack of information regarding their arrest and court proceedings, and insecurity about the future. In contrast, sentenced prisoners are usually older (over thirty-five), and more likely to be violent offenders. They frequently engage in conflicts at their institutions or have a conflict or a breakup with family members. The sentenced prisoners experience loss of social freedom, family support, fear of physical or sexual violence in the institution, and incarceration's added stress. These dynamic risk factors have a greater influence on their decision to attempt suicide.[9]

PRIOR SUICIDE ATTEMPT

A prior near-lethal suicide attempt such as attempted hanging or overdose is the single most common predictor of suicide. Death occurs four times more often among attempters than among non-attempters, and most occur less than four years after the near-lethal attempt.[15] The predictors of suicide among attempters who eventually kill themselves include repeated attempts, the lethality of method, and mental illness such as depression and severe anxiety. Therefore, incarcerated previous attempters form a well-defined high-risk group.

In a comprehensive review of near-lethal suicide attempts by persons involved in the criminal justice process in England and Wales, Marzano et al.[16] identified deficiencies in risk assessment as a critical issue. Placing a near-lethal suicide attempter in the risk management "document" decreases the chance of suicide. Marzano et al. further noted a strong association between near-lethal self-harm and mental disorders. This underscores the importance of screening for mental disorder and suicidality at the earliest point in the criminal justice pathway.

Past near-lethal suicide attempt by hanging or overdose is associated with high suicide intent.[16, 11] Inmates who enter the system with such a history are likely to act on their intent in the early stages of incarceration, indicating a strong need for systematic suicide screening at booking into jails and reception at prisons.

INITIAL VS. SUBSEQUENT ARREST

First-time arrestees' rate of suicide is seven times higher than those who have had prior arrests.[13] The often-cited reason for such a high rate compared with prior arrestees is "the shock of first confinement," in which inmates acutely experience the deprivation of normal status due to loss of a job, dignity, and social connections. Compared with jails, prisons have a lower suicide rate. That's because most convicted persons enter prisons after being screened and having their potential risk identified and mitigated. So their profile is known before they enter prisons. Furthermore, most prisons have a well-established protocol to screen and identify those at risk, though the suicide rate in prisons is higher than in the general U.S. population.

The prospect of receiving a harsh, lengthy sentence, particularly for young adults, persons with no history of prior crime, or persons in good standing in the community, is highly correlated with increased suicide risk. Suicide notes commonly address the anguish and pain at the prospect of a lengthy sentence.

COURT PROCEEDINGS

New charges, unanticipated harsh sentences, and the loss of appeal pose a high suicide risk. The period immediately after the court proceedings is especially problematic. Often, a sentence the inmate believes he or she does not deserve is a significant factor that leads to feelings of hopelessness. Some correctional programs prepare inmates who face a new sentencing for a negative outcome and provide counseling to them before and after court proceedings.

ADMINISTRATIVE SEGREGATION

Prisoners held in isolation or administrative segregation have a higher risk of suicide. Solitary isolation is a common factor in suicide, irrespective of the type of facility. Jail and prison inmates in solitary confinement spend approximately twenty-three hours alone. Such isolation causes sensory deprivation, a factor that contributes to extreme stress and confusion. Inmates placed in administrative segregation are at risk of developing a new mental disorder or deterioration of an already present mental disorder.

If placed in solitary confinement, psychotic inmates may become more delusional and hallucinatory, and they lose touch with reality. Depressed inmates with hopelessness who are left alone are at higher risk than those with depression alone. Many suicides occur when prisoners are alone, even if they are technically sharing a cell.[3] A study of suicide in Belgium prisons by Favrile et al. found that 63% of suicides occurred when cellmates were out of the cell, and only 24% occurred in shared cells.[17] When inmates are in sight of staff members or other inmates, the likelihood of suicide is remote.

Correctional officers may leave an arrestee unattended in a single cell while completing the customary paperwork. Many attempted or completed suicides occur during the first few hours of detention. Most suicides by hanging occur in isolation in a single cell or when a detainee is left alone.

Lifers have a higher suicide risk,[18] and suicide vulnerability increases with the length of sentence.[19]

LOSSES AND ADJUSTMENT PROBLEMS

The recent loss of stabilizing influence, such as the death of a mother, father, wife, husband, boyfriend, or girlfriend—or any bad news—may precipitate suicide in vulnerable individuals. The threat or actual loss of custody of children is reflected in the history of a few completed suicides. Financial loss and the recent loss of job, poor health, or a terminal illness were some other precipitants.

Severe guilt or shame over the offense is a significant factor, especially for those charged with or sentenced for sex offenses. Same-sex rape or threat of rape is another precipitant. A long-term inmate may experience intense anxiety at the time of impending release due to the difficulty in adjusting to society and lack of support system, employment, or trade skills. Abrupt discontinuation of psychiatric medication (loss of ability to continue medications) at entry into detention may frustrate a mentally ill detainee.

Unemployment [20] is linked to an elevated risk of suicide. Occupational social class, suicide, and deliberate self-harm (DSH) are inversely linked: the lower the social class, the higher the risk of suicidal behavior.

MENTAL DISORDERS AS A RISK FACTOR

About 16%–20% of the incarcerated population in the United States have serious mental illnesses, including schizophrenia, bipolar disorder or other psychotic disorders, major depression, and PTSD. Another 25% have anxiety disorders, adjustment disorders, obsessive-compulsive disorder, and organic mental disorders. The onset of the psychiatric disorder may happen before or during incarceration, with most pre-incarceration diagnoses having an onset before age eighteen. Inmates' criminal profiles show that a substantial number have a personality disorder, including borderline personality disorder and antisocial personality disorder.

According to a study by the U.S. Department of Justice,[21] over 50% of all prison and jail inmates have a mental health problem, compared with 11% in the general U.S. population, yet only one-third receive minimum psychiatric care.

Similar trends have been observed in non-U.S. populations. A review of mental health services in the Canadian correctional system shows that 15%–20% of prison inmates have a serious mental illness, consistent with the U.S.

inmate population.[22] Fazel and Seewald's comprehensive meta-analysis of 33,588 seriously mentally ill prisoners in 24 countries in 2012 shows that 3.6% had psychotic illnesses among male prisoners, and 10.2% had major depression. The prevalence rates among women were 3.9% and 14.1%, respectively.[23] The proportion was even higher in maximum-security prisons.[14]

For patients with first-episode schizophrenia, though more at risk than chronic patients, hallucinations and delusions are protective, except for command hallucinations.[10]

It is common for inmates to have multiple psychiatric disorders with comorbid substance abuse. In a 1988 study by Daniel, Robins, and Reid,[24] 90% of consecutively admitted female prisoners had an Axis I clinical psychiatric disorder, and 67% had more than one disorder. In a study of 1,272 female arrestees in Cook County, Illinois, 80% had one or more lifetime psychiatric disorders.[25]

A systematic review of 62 surveys of the incarcerated population, including 23,000 prisoners from twelve Western countries[26], showed that among men, 3.7% had a psychotic illness, 10% had major depression, and 65% had a personality disorder, including 47% with an antisocial personality disorder. Among women, 4% had psychosis, 12% had major depression, and 42% had a personality disorder. Also, a significant number suffered from anxiety disorders, including PTSD, organic disorders, short- and long-term sequelae of traumatic brain injury (TBI), suicidal behaviors, distress associated with all forms of abuse, ADHD, and other developmental disorders, including mental retardation and Asperger's disorder.

Mood Disorders

Inmates diagnosed with mood disorders, including major depressive disorder, unspecified depressive disorder, and bipolar disorder are at higher risk for suicide than those diagnosed with any other diagnostic categories. The high risk is consistent with the general community for this diagnostic category. Twenty-five to sixty percent of patients with bipolar disorder will attempt suicide at least once in their lifetime, while between 4% and 19% will commit suicide.

McLean et al.[20] noted that suicide risk appears to be elevated around the time of the first diagnosis. For those with bipolar disorder and schizophrenia, the elevated risk for suicide is further exacerbated by other risk factors, including a history of suicide attempts, and other comorbid psychiatric diagnoses, such as impulse control disorder, ADHD, drug or alcohol misuse, anxiety, recent bereavement, and hopelessness.

Depressive disorders are more often linked to suicide than to any other psychiatric illness. Specific characteristics of mood disorders that are correlated with suicide include the first episode of depression, active psychiatric treatment, and medication use at the time of entry to jail or prison.

Depression and hopelessness appear to be the two most common mental states at the time of a suicidal act.[27] Although depression and suicide co-occur, hopelessness and suicide have a stronger correlation than do depression and suicide. Negative life events and sentence length indirectly impact suicidality by affecting depression. Using a multivariate model to predict suicide by inmates, Ivanoff and Jang[28] studied the relationship among depression, hopelessness, suicidality, and social desirability. They found that negative life events and sentence length indirectly impact suicidality by causing depression. Inmates with higher social desirability had lower levels of depression; thus, they had lower suicidality levels.

Anxiety Disorders

Anxiety experienced by inmates at various times of incarceration, particularly on entry into the system or just before release, may act as a risk factor. Anxiety symptoms mixed with agitation, depression, and hopelessness further increase the risk.

Personality Disorders and Traits

There may be increased suicide risk associated with individual/personality factors. The evidence is inconclusive.[20] Nevertheless, it can be stated with reasonable confidence that suicide risk is higher in a wide range of personality traits, including hopelessness, neuroticism, extroversion, impulsivity, aggression, anger, irritability, and hostility.[20]

Although antisocial personality disorder is "endemic to correctional settings",[29] the relationship between antisocial personality disorder and suicide risk seems inconclusive. Only one study found a positive correlation between the two. Verona et al.[30] used the Psychopathy Checklist-Revised (PCL-R) to study 313 male inmates in a federal institution in Florida. They found a positive correlation between antisocial deviance and suicidal tendencies in male inmates.

Borderline personality disorder (BPD) increases the risk for suicide attempts and completion due to poor interpersonal skills, impulsivity, and affective instability. In prison, impulsivity can be a factor in young prisoners with BPD and depressive disorders and in those who are victims of cluster suicides. Although a direct link between impulsivity and suicide cannot be established, only a few engage in careful preparation during days preceding the suicide.[31]

Substance Use Disorders (SUDs)

Almost 70% of the incarcerated population have a history of substance abuse, which may or may not be related to their criminal behavior. The World Health Organization (WHO) Task Force* identified substance abuse as a risk factor for suicide.[32] Alcohol intoxication and withdrawal is a known factor for suicides in jails. In a study of suicides in jails and lockups, Hayes found that 20% who died by suicide were intoxicated at the time of their detention.[33]

Timeframes of substance withdrawal offer a critical window for prevention efforts. Alcohol withdrawal-related suicide occurs during the first seventy-two hours, while opiate withdrawal-related suicide occurs within three to seven days.[34] Benzodiazepine withdrawal, coupled with rebound anxiety commonly found from seven to fourteen days after the cessation, may act as a precipitant to suicidal thinking in certain inmates. However, abrupt discontinuation of even high doses does not precipitate suicidal ideation or behaviors. More often, during the initial stages of benzodiazepine therapy, some patients may experience suicidal ideation.[35]

Substance misuse increases the risk of suicide attempts and death by suicide. The risk associated with opioid use disorders and mixed intravenous drug use is greater than that for alcohol misuse. Impulsive suicide attempts under intoxication are more common among arrestees than people in the community.[6]

Intermittent suicidal thinking is observed among incarcerated drug abusers due to forced abstinence and undeveloped coping skills because of years of dependency. The risk of suicide is highest among opiate users who also have psychiatric disorders.[36]

Post-Traumatic Stress Disorder

Exposure to specific and cumulative trauma is a common finding among the incarcerated population. About 6% of men and 21% of women in prisons have lifetime exposure to high levels of trauma during childhood and later in life. [37]

The trauma is usually related to physical abuse, sexual abuse, and assaults—including rape, domestic violence, prison rape, harassment, and bullying. Veterans in jails and prisons report a significant exposure to combat trauma in the war zones of Afghanistan, Iraq, and other deployments.

Exposure to trauma causes PTSD in vulnerable people, depending on the severity and the duration of the traumatic experience. PTSD is diagnosed when a person exposed to a single or cumulative trauma reports having symptoms of reliving trauma with nightmares and intrusive recollections, flashbacks, and hyperarousal, including startle reaction, panic attacks, severe anxiety, and hypervigilance. These symptoms lead to psychosocial dysfunction, including alcohol dependence, substance abuse, and criminal behaviors. PTSD in prisons and jails is often underdiagnosed and untreated.

A significant association exists between suicidality and PTSD. More often, PTSD is linked to aggressive behaviors, impulsivity, and criminal behaviors in the community and military population, with a stronger association in men.

In New Zealand, Favril et al. (2020)[38] found that prisoners with PTSD and substance abuse were at higher risk for suicide ideation than persons without PTSD. The correlation between suicidal ideation and suicide acts *and* PTSD and substance use disorders can be due to poor impulse control from substance abuse. Reliving trauma can cause suicidal ideation, which may progress to suicidal acts and behaviors.

Traumatic Brain Injury (TBI) and Mild Cognitive Impairment (MCI)
The Centers for Disease Control (CDC) recognizes that traumatic brain injury is a significant problem in the incarcerated population. Studies have indicated that 25%–87% of inmates have sustained at least one head injury during their lifetime. Prisoners who have experienced head injuries tend to suffer from depression, anxiety, substance abuse, and suicidal ideation and behaviors. Interestingly, women who were convicted of a violent crime often have a history of prior TBI.[39] Many women with substance abuse also have a history of TBI.

Concussions and TBI can produce mild cognitive impairment manifested by executive function deficits, language difficulties, short-term memory deficits, delayed recall problems, attention deficit, anger control problems, impulsivity, and slowed verbal and physical responses. Some inmates may show suicidal behaviors when they become frustrated with jails and prisons' rigid environment and rules.

Mental health providers and medical staff should gather a history of head injuries and inmates' concussions during routine evaluations. A screening instrument such as the Mini-Mental Status Examination (MMSE) or Montreal Cognitive Assessment (MOCA) is easy to administer to identify mild cognitive impairment. These instruments assess executive functioning, attention, language, short-term memory, delayed recall, and orientation.

Chronic Physical Conditions

Chronic and intractable medical conditions, severe and persistent pain, terminal cancer, and HIV/AIDS are moderately correlated with risk of suicide.

PROTECTIVE FACTORS

1. Ability to identify the reason for living
2. Problem-solving skills
3. Religious beliefs against suicide and personal faith in God or a higher power
4. Social support in the institution
5. Family support
6. Lack of suicidal ideation
7. View of death as negative
8. Willingness to engage with peers and staff
9. Actively seeking mental health treatment

Protective factors counterbalance risk factors. They include positive social support, a sense of responsibility, family connectedness, children at home, spirituality and faith, reality testing ability, positive therapeutic relationship, coping skills, and problem-solving skills. McLean et al.[20] reported that marriage in the U.S. is a protective factor against suicide, more so for White females than Black females. Marriage has a "buffering effect" against socio-economic inequalities related to suicide, particularly for men. Social support, in general, is protective against suicide among a range of population groups, including Black Americans and women who have experienced domestic abuse.

SUICIDE RISK ASSESSMENT PROCESS

Knowledge of risk and protective factors does not necessarily lead to an adequate assessment of an inmate at risk, but it is the starting point in the assessment process. No standardized assessment tool exists, though clinicians use tests such as the Beck Scale for Suicidal Ideation, the Brief Reasons for Living Inventory, the Suicide Probability Scale, and the SAD PERSONS scale. But none of them are corrections specific. No state administrative codes specify the details of risk assessment procedures, except to stipulate that there must be a suicide risk assessment completed on inmates at risk.

Suicide risk assessment in the correctional setting must be done at every stage of incarceration from booking to release. A reliable suicide risk assessment consists of the following procedures:

1. Suicide screening at booking
2. Risk assessment clinical interview
3. Risk analysis
4. Risk reassessment

Screening

While a simple self-report scale can be used to identify inmates with suicidal ideation,[40] such self-reports are deceptive.[11] Time and again, inmates conceal their true intent.

One of the commonly used screening tools in outpatient and crisis situations is the Columbia-Suicide Severity Rating Scale (C-SSRS). The scale focuses on suicide ideation and behaviors. The scale consists of six Yes or No questions. A respondent is asked about suicidal thoughts, feeling toward suicide, and suicidal behaviors during the past three months and their lifetime.

Question 1 focuses on the respondent's wish to be dead

Question 2 involves non-specific suicidal thoughts

Questions 3 elicits current active suicide ideation without intent to act

Question 4 elicits active suicide ideation with some intent to act without a specific plan

Question 5 addresses the presence of current active suicidal ideation with a specific plan and intent

Question 6 addresses suicide behavior over a lifetime and during the past three months

If the respondent answers yes to question #1, he/she is asked to skip Question #2 and proceed to Questions 3 to 5. If he/she answers no, they are asked to skip to Question #6. If the answer to any of the six questions is yes, a referral to a mental health professional is indicated. A "yes" answer to Questions 4, 5, or 6 indicates high risk.

Though it is a valid and reliable rating scale to assess suicide risk, the scale's suitability in correctional settings is questionable because the scale does not consider any corrections-specific risk factors or the setting.

Although the effectiveness of suicide screening instruments and checklists are not strong due to high false positives and false negatives,[41] their use is considered important for any suicide prevention program.

Suicide Screening Tool

A screening tool consistent with the known risk factors of suicide in jails and prisons is likely to identify most inmates at risk—but not necessarily everyone at risk because an inmate's risk changes over time. Yet research and clinical experience have established distinct and specific risk factors for inmates.

Known risk factors that increase the likelihood of suicide:

1. Prior near-lethal suicide attempt
2. Current suicidal ideation, plan, and intent
3. Recent psychosocial stressors
4. Availability of means: rope, anchor points, drugs
5. Prior psychiatric hospitalization and medication use
6. Mood disorders; depressive disorders
7. Chronic intractable pain and other chronic disabling physical conditions
8. Psychological states of hopelessness, guilt, anxiety, agitation, insomnia, or a feeling of being trapped
9. Psychiatric disorders with comorbid substance abuse
10. Alcohol and opiate intoxication
11. A charge involving a shocking crime

Proposed Screening Questionnaire and Observations

Based on the known factors that increase the likelihood of suicide, a useful screening questionnaire is proposed below. The questionnaire should be administered at booking by a mental health professional or a trained correctional officer.

1. Is the detainee thinking about harming him/herself?

2. Does the arresting officer believe that the detainee may take his or her life?
3. Does the detainee have a psychiatric/mental health history, including psychotropic medication use?
4. Has the detainee made a previous near-lethal suicide attempt during the preceding twelve months?
5. Does the detainee have a history of drug or alcohol abuse?
6. Is the detainee intoxicated with alcohol or drugs at the time of booking?
7. Does the detainee lack close family or friends in the community?
8. Has the detainee experienced a significant loss within the last six months?
9. Does the detainee hold a position of respect in the community?
10. Is the detainee accused of or charged with a shocking crime?
11. Is the detainee suffering from acute pain or a chronic intractable medical condition?
12. Is the detainee feeling helpless, hopeless, anxious, agitated, or trapped?
13. Does the detainee appear to be depressed, sad, or guilt-ridden?

Each question should have a provision to mark yes or no and explain. Questions concerning current positive suicidal ideation and past near-lethal attempts within a year should be given more weight in assessing an inmate's potential risk. The arresting officer's feeling, though subjective, must be given careful consideration.

Risk Assessment Interview

The risk assessment clinical interview and a mental status examination are conducted after a referral from an intake worker or a correctional officer who suspects an inmate is at risk. Also, critical risk factors identified in the suicide screening questionnaire set the required clinical interview in motion.

A qualified mental health professional, including a licensed professional counselor, social worker, psychologist, or a psychiatrist must conduct the interview. At the outset of the clinical interview, the evaluator must gather information from the correctional officer or any person who placed the inmate on suicide watch. It is unusual for a mental health professional to contact a family member, but any information received by the jailers from a family member and their observations of the inmate must be shared with the evaluator. Obligatory sharing of information by the correctional officer with the mental health professional fulfills the staff's collective responsibility, specifically in identifying an inmate at risk, because the officers are tasked to monitor inmates under suicide watch.

The interview is preferably conducted in a semi-structured format[42] to comport with psychiatric disorders and mental state correlated with suicide risk. It usually takes about thirty to forty minutes. During the interview, it is appropriate to ask direct questions without being judgmental about suicidal ideation, intent, and plan. Questions should focus on the following:

1. Is the inmate entertaining suicidal ideation?
2. Does the inmate have a plan and intent to harm him/herself?

3. Has the inmate made any previous suicide attempt, and if so, what was the nature of the attempt?
4. Is the inmate apprehensive about problems other than the current situation?
5. Does the inmate feel helpless, hopeless, or that he/she has nothing to look forward to?
6. Does the inmate show signs of depression such as crying, social withdrawal, emotional flatness, emotional over-activity, or depressed mood?
7. Is the inmate overly anxious, afraid, or angry?
8. Does the inmate feel unusually embarrassed or ashamed of the situation?
9. Does the inmate act strangely?
10. Does the inmate appear under the influence of drugs or alcohol?
11. Does the inmate show signs of withdrawal from drugs?
12. Does the inmate suffer from a depressive, anxiety, or psychotic disorder?
13. Does the inmate have symptoms of PTSD?
14. Does the inmate have adequate coping and cognitive resources?
15. Does the inmate have an adequate support system?

Risk Analysis

The final step in suicide risk assessment is the risk analysis—the process with which the evaluator or the treatment team, if any, synthesizes all the relevant static and dynamic risk factors and protective factors, including the relevant data from the screening questionnaire and clinical interview. The evaluator must check the consistency of the information across the data gathering process. Any inconsistency between the denial and behavior pattern may raise questions on suicidal ideation and the behaviors' veracity.

Individuals who deny a present intention to end their lives are often still at high risk for suicide.[43] Inmates who are committed to ending their lives do not want to be stopped. Often, they do not want to be ostracized by other inmates, and would be unhappy about the punitive measure if they are placed on suicide precautions. Therefore, clinicians are cautioned not to rely exclusively on the direct statements of an inmate who denies that he/she has suicidal ideation or a history of past suicidal behaviors. In this context, it is imperative that a comprehensive suicide risk assessment of all risk and protective factors be performed.

The risk analysis allows the determination of the level of supervision, clinical and custodial monitoring needs, and treatment needs of those identified as at risk. The level of the watch can be on a continuum of the constant watch, intermittent watch every 15 minutes to suicide observation every 30 minutes to transfer to release to the general population. Based on the analysis, the mental health professional decides to keep an inmate on suicide watch until their risk mitigates or releases them from the watch and transfers the inmate out of the observation cell to the general prison population.

The evaluator must document the findings of the clinical interview and risk analysis promptly.

Risk Reassessment
Changing situations and factors affect an inmate's risk, even among those who received the appropriate intervention.

Adjustment to a new institution after a transfer and non-prison-related factors may affect an inmate. Times of bereavement, new court hearings, and denial of a bond leave detainees particularly vulnerable. In such situations, a new risk assessment is indicated. Repeat risk assessment after the first month following prison arrival should also be considered. Marzano et al.[16] found that three-quarters of men and women in the Oxford studies of near-fatal self-harm had carried out their attempts over a month after their first reception into custody.

In many jails and prisons, "recyclers" or "frequent flyers" are common. A few have suicidal tendencies. They must also receive a risk assessment when they are readmitted. A master list of inmates who were placed on suicide watch during incarceration will facilitate easy identification when they return to the facility. An electronic "suicide alert" in the individual private screen of a previously suicidal inmate will alert the mental health professional who must review his/her previous records before conducting a suicide risk assessment. A prior serious suicide attempt may serve as a marker for future identification of potential future attempts.

Those who are placed on suicide watch must receive a daily suicide risk assessment until their risk no longer exists. Any inmate who is newly placed in solitary confinement must receive regular mental health assessment, possibly weekly, and careful consideration must be given for a full suicide risk assessment. Thus, a comprehensive suicide risk assessment as outlined earlier must be an essential component of suicide prevention programs in jails and prisons.

Telepsychiatry

A word about telehealth assessment is appropriate because of the changing health care environment due to the COVID-19 pandemic. Telepsychiatry has been initiated at many facilities recently. Generally, tele-mental health assessments and medication monitoring are reserved for inmates who are relatively stable on psychotropic medications. Inmates for the telehealth services are selected based on diagnosis, class of psychotropic medications, and absence of problematic and suicidal behaviors. Assessment and monitoring are done using electronic medical records (EMR). The psychiatrist trained in using telepsychiatry sees the inmate/patients every ninety days to assess their stability and renew their medications.

For suicide risk assessment, a face-to-face interview and mental health assessment are preferred because of the importance of observing the inmate in his/her environment and the need to gather information from the officers and issuing directions for supervision.

CONCLUSION

Using a reliable suicide screening instrument is the first step toward identification of at-risk inmates. Beyond screening, timely and systematic suicide risk assessment is the next step in triaging, monitoring, and preventive intervention efforts.

REFERENCES

1. Estelle v. Gamble, 429 US 97 (1976)
2. Mental Health Screening and Evaluation, National Commission on Correctional Health Care, Standard JE-05 (2020)

3. Hayes, L and Hayes, MS. *National and State Standards for Prison Suicide Prevention: A Report Card.* Journal of Correctional Health Care 3(1) (1996) 5–38

4. Daniel, AE. *Preventing suicide in prison: a collaborative responsibility of administrative, custodial, and clinical staff.* Journal of the American Academy of Psychiatry and the Law 34(2) (2006) 165–175

5. Kline-Simon, AH, Sterling, S, Young-Wolff K, et al. *Estimates of Workload Associated With Suicide Risk Alerts After Implementation of Risk-Prediction Model.* JAMA Netw Open 3(10) (2020) e2021189

6. Simon, RI. *Suicide risk assessment: What is the standard of care?* Journal of American Academy of Psychiatry and the Law 30(3) (2002) 340–344

7. Estate of Kempf v. Washington City, No. CV.15-1125, 2018 WL4354547

8. Palakovic v. Wetzel, 854 F.3d 209 (3d Cir. 2017)

9. Konrad, N, Daigle, MS, Daniel, AE, Dear, GE, Frottier P, Hayes. LM, Kerkhof, A, Liebling, A, Sarchiapone, M: (2007) *Preventing suicide in prisons, part I. Recommendations from the International Association for Suicide Prevention Task Force on Suicide in Prisons.* CRISIS 28 (3) (2007) 113–121

10. Nordentorf, M. *Prevention of suicide and attempted suicide in Denmark. epidemiological studies of suicide and intervention studies in selected risk groups,* Danish Medical Bulletin 54(4) (2007) 306–69

11. Daniel, AE and Fleming J. *Suicides in a state correctional system 1992–2002: A Review.* Journal of Correctional Health Care 12 (1) (2006) 24–35

12. Bureau of Justice Statistics, Deaths in Custody Reporting Program and Centers for Disease Control and Prevention (2015)

13. Bureau of Justice Statistics, Deaths in Custody Reporting Program and Centers for Disease Control and Prevention (2016)

14. Lester, D and Danto, BL. *Suicide Behind Bars: Prediction and Prevention. Philadelphia: The Charles Press* (1993)18–21

15. Christensen, E, et al. *Risk of repetition of suicide attempt, suicide, or all deaths after an episode of attempted suicide: a register-based survival analysis.* Aust NZ Journal of psychiatry 41(3) (2007) 257–65

16. Marzano, L, Hawton, K, Rivlin, A, et al. *An Overview of Initiatives Based on a Systematic Review of Research on Near-Lethal Suicide Attempts, Prevention of Suicidal Behavior in Prisons.* CRISIS 37(5) (2016) 323–334

17. Favril, L, Wittouck, C, Audenaert, K and Vander Laenen, F. *A 17-Year National Study of Prison Suicides in Belgium.* CRISIS 40(1) (2019) 42–53

18. Liebling, A. *Role of the prison environment in prison suicide and prisoner distress,* In G.E. Dear (ed) *Preventing suicide and other self-harm in prison (2006) 16–28 Basing-Stoke: UK Palgrave-McMillan*

19. Frottier, P, Frühwald, S, Ritter, K, Eher, R, Schwärzler, J and Bauer P. *Jailhouse Blues revisited.* Soc Psychiatry Psychiatr Epidemiol 37(2) (2002) 68–73

20. McLean, J, Maxwell, M, Platt, S, Harris, F and Jepson, R. *Risk and Protective Factors for Suicide and Suicidal*

Behavior: A Literature Review. Social Research, Scottish Government (2008)

21. James, DJ and Glaze LE. *Mental Health Problems of Prison and Jail Inmates.* Department of Justice, Washington DC, Bureau of Justice Statistics Special Report, September 2006

22. Simpson, AI, McMaster, JJ and Cohen, SN. *Challenges for Canada in meeting the needs of persons with serious mental illness in prison.* Journal of American Academy of Psychiatry and the Law 41(4) (2013) 501

23. Fazel, S and Seewald, K. *Severe Mental Illness in 33,588 Prisoners Worldwide: Systematic Review and Meta-Regression Analysis.* British Journal of Psychiatry 200 (5) (2012) 364–73

24. Daniel, AE, Robins, AJ, Reid, JC and Wilfley, DE. *Lifetime and six-month prevalence of psychiatric disorders among sentenced female offenders.* Bulletin of American Academy of Psychiatry and the Law 16(4) (1988) 333–42

25. Teplin, LA, Abram, KM and McClelland, GM. *Prevalence of psychiatric disorders among incarcerated women: Pretrial jail detainees.* Archives of General Psychiatry 53 (1996) 505–12

26. Fazel, S and Danesh, J. *Serious Mental Disorder in 23,000 prisoners: A systematic review of 62 surveys,* The Lancet 359 (9306) (2002) 545–550

27. Redding, RE. *Depression in jailed women defendants and its relationship to their adjudicative competence.* Journal of American Academy of Psychiatry and the Law 25 (1997) 105–19

28. Ivanoff, A and Jang, SJ. *The role of hopelessness and social desirability in predicting suicidal behavior: a study of prison inmates.* Journal of Consulting and Clinical Psychology 59 (1991)394–9

29. Trestman, RL. *Behind Bars: Personality Disorders.* Journal of American Academy of Psychiatry and the Law 28 (2000) 232–5

30. Verona, E, Patrick, CJ and Joiner, TE. *Psychopathy, anti-social personality, and suicide risk.* Journal of Abnormal Psychology 110 (2001) 462–70

31. Kerkhof, AJ and Bernasco, W. *Suicidal behavior in jails and prisons in the Netherlands: incidence, characteristics, and prevention.* Suicide Life Threat Behavior 20 (1990) 123–37

32. WHO Resource Guide Update (2007) Preventing Suicide in Jails and Prisons

33. Hayes, L. *National Study of Jail Suicide 20 Years Later,* Washington DC, U.S. Department of Justice, National Institute of Justice (2010)

34. FDA: Clonazepam: www.accessdata.fda.gov

35. Felthous, AR. *Preventing Jailhouse Suicides.* Bulletin of American Academy of Psychiatry and the Law 22 (1994) 477–88

36. Kokkevi, A, and Stefanis, C. *Drug abuse and psychiatric comorbidity.* Comprehensive Psychiatry 36 (1995) 329–37

37. Facer-Irwin, E, Blackwood, NJ, Bird, A, Dickson, H et al. *PTSD in prison settings: A systematic review and met-analysis of comorbid mental disorders and problematic behaviors* (2019) www. Ncbi.nlm.nih.gov

38. Favril, L, Devon, I, Gear, C and Wilhelm K. (2020) *Mental disorders and risk of suicide attempt in prisoners.* Social Psychiatry and Psychiatric Epidemiology, 55 (9) (2020) 11

39. Brewer Smyth, K, Burgess, AW and Shults J. *Physical and sexual abuse, salivary cortical, and neurologic correlates of violent criminal behavior in female prison inmates.* Biological Psychiatry 55 (1) (2004) 21–31

40. Bonner, RL and Rich, AR. *Psychosocial Vulnerability, Life Stress, And Suicidal Ideation in a Jail Population, A Cross-validation,* Suicide and Life-Threatening Behavior 20 (1990) 220–234

41. O'Connor, E, Gaynes, B, Burda, B, Williams, C and Whitlock, E. *AHRQ Screening for Suicide Risk in Primary Care: A Systematic Evidence Review.* U.S. Preventive Services Task Force Publication (2013) 13-05188-EF-1

42. Carlson. DK, *The Jail Suicide Assessment Tool (JSAT)* https://www.usmarshals.gov/prisoner/assessment _tool.pdf

43. Hayes, L. *Suicide Prevention in Correctional Facilities: Reflections and Next Steps.,* International Journal of Law and Psychiatry 36 (2013) 188–184

* In recognition of suicide as a global problem, the World Health Organization (WHO) assembled a group of experts to study the incidence and prevalence of suicide and the risk factors and recommendations for preventing and managing suicidal inmates. In 2000, WHO published its first report: "A Resource Guide to Prevent Suicide in Jails and Prisons." Seven distinguished researchers and I updated The Resource Guide in 2006 for jails and prisons in two separate reports.

The members included Norbert Konrad, MD (Germany); Marc Daigle, PhD (Canada); Greg Dear, PhD (Australia); Patrick Frottier, MD (Austria); Lindsay M. Hayes (United States); Ad Kerkoff, PhD (The Netherlands); Alison Liebling, PhD (UK); Marco Sarchiapone, MD (Italy); and Anasseril E. Daniel, MD (United States).

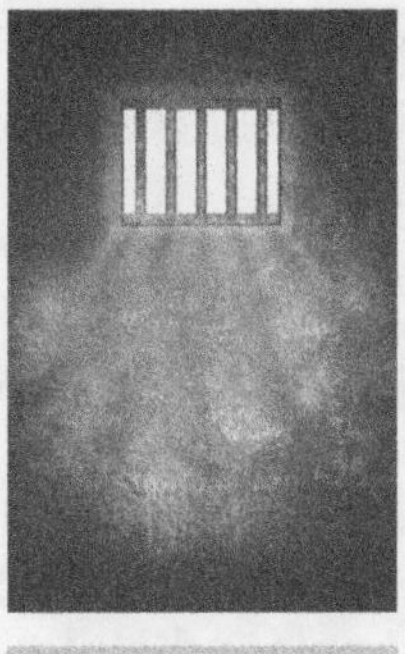

CHAPTER 4

SUICIDE PREVENTION PROGRAM: POLICIES, PROCEDURES, AND PRACTICES

In a Federal lawsuit claiming malpractice and deliberate indifference, Correctional Medical Services, a private health-care agency, was found liable because of noncompliance with the written institutional policy on suicide prevention by its professional staff (*Woodward v. Correctional Medical Services*).[1] Justin Farver, a twenty-three-year-old male with cerebral palsy, hanged himself with a sheet in Lake County Jail in Waukegan, Illinois, on October 13, 1998, three weeks after his detention. At intake screening, he reported a history of depression, bipolar disorder, past multiple suicide attempts, and suicidal ideation. The nurse who conducted the screening documented that Farver expressed thoughts of killing himself; however, she did not notify the shift commander, though the jail policy required her to do so.

On October 1, a social worker evaluated and documented that Farver had an extensive history of suicide attempts and several suicide risk factors. He further noted that Farver had "suicidal proclivities," but took no action to place him on suicide watch, believing that Farver was already on watch because he was in the medical unit.

The jail psychiatrist evaluated Farver on October 11. He found him feeling "hopeless, helpless, and worthless" and prescribed Zoloft and Ativan. He, too, incorrectly believed that Mr. Farver was on suicide watch.

The family filed a §1983 claim against Lake County's sheriff, the social worker, the psychiatrist, and the company providing health-care services. They also filed an Illinois wrongful death claim against the social worker and the psychiatrist.

In May 2001, in denying a summary judgment motion by the defendants, the judge concluded that a reasonable jury would find that the social worker and the psychiatrist acted with deliberate indifference to a substantial and obvious risk that Farver would take his life. Following the judge's opinion and order, the family settled the case against the Lake County sheriff before the trial involving the health-care providers and the health services company.

During the trial in 2002, two experts testified that failure to alert the shift commander was a deviation from the National Commission on Correctional Health Care (NCCHC) standard. The expert further testified that the health services provider at the jail failed to follow its policies and procedures. The jury found that the nurse and the psychiatrist were not liable for Farver's death, while the social worker and the health services provider were liable. In this trial, the plaintiff showed that the staff did not follow the health-care company's published policies and that the team routinely violated its policies regarding intake, screening, and precautions.

Suicide prevention is not carried out uniformly in jails and prisons. A wide variation exists in program implementation from jail to jail and prison to prison. Many facilities are satisfied with developing policies and procedures, placing undue emphasis on screening instruments, and having a "spot check mentality," rather than performing a comprehensive suicide risk assessment. It is commonly assumed that a reduced suicide rate from the national or regional level, or even from the former level in the same institution, is all that can be achieved.

A fully implemented 24/7 suicide prevention program not only saves lives but also is the best defense against liability claims. Some lawsuits allege that policies, customs, and practices directly cause or contribute to an inmate's wrongful death. This type of claim had its roots in *Monell v. Department of Social Services* (1978).[2] In this case, the U.S. Supreme Court held that "municipal entities may be sued for constitutional deprivations visited under a governmental 'custom' even though such a custom has not received formal approval through the body's official decision-making channels."

Suicide prevention is a collaborative responsibility.[3] The medical and mental health staff, administration, and correctional officers have specific roles in keeping the inmates safe. Mental health professionals perform the risk assessment, mental health evaluation, medication management, and mental health review of inmates in administrative segregation and crisis management. The correctional officers conduct the initial screening and monitor the inmate on watch. Administration provides the facility's structure and organization and is responsible for creating an attitude among the staff that suicides can and should be prevented. The medical staff performs the physical assessment, chronic care, and emergency management, including care after an inmate's hanging. The correctional officers observe any changes in behaviors and obvious mental symptoms, report them to mental health providers, and conduct suicide watch and monitoring. Compartmentalization of responsibilities is the norm, yet the staff must all work together.

A comprehensive suicide prevention program aims to provide correctional officers and health-care professionals with guidelines to recognize inmates' mental health needs and suicidal tendencies, correctly classify and house the mentally ill and suicidal inmates, and document all interventions and treatment.[4]

The strength and effectiveness of a suicide prevention program depends on three components. They include:

1. policies;
2. procedures; and
3. practices.

POLICIES

Policies must be concise and adequate to meet the mission and objectives and must include specific procedures needed to meet these objectives. How a policy is adhered to determines the outcome of any lawsuit claiming that a "custom and practice" at that facility caused or contributed to a wrongful death.

Suppose a facility policy states that upon determination of suicide risk of an inmate, reasonable measures must be taken to prevent the inmate from attempting or completing suicide and that the inmate should be referred to medical or mental health professionals for evaluation and appropriate intervention. Noncompliance with any step during the process from screening to referral may be construed as a deviation from the established facility policy. Suppose the practice of a 15-minute suicide watch is not uniformly carried out as prescribed in the written policy at an institution. In that case, it can be conceived as lack of supervision and monitoring of an inmate on suicide watch. The non-adherence with the written policy would imply that the custom and practice had a direct and proximate role in causing an inmate's wrongful death. Similarly, if officers, while performing suicide watch, routinely walk by the cell without looking into the cell, making sure the inmate is "alive and breathing," such a practice may be viewed as a "custom," not approved by the facility, contributing to an inmate's death.

Suicide prevention is more than staff education. It is built upon interrelated policies including, but not limited to, access to mental health care, suicide prevention measures, psychotropic medications, involuntary medications, and treatment of mentally ill inmates. All policies and procedures should be written to prevent suicides, meet the standard of care, and avoid deliberate indifference claims.

Access to Mental Health Care

Access to mental health services by inmates is a significant component of a comprehensive suicide prevention program. Almost 50% of inmates who intend to seriously harm themselves contact mental health providers before their attempts.[5]

The NCCHC standard[4] states that "access to care means that in a timely manner a patient (inmate) can be seen by a clinician and be given professional clinical judgment and receive care that is ordered." Mental health services broadly include a range of diagnostic, treatment, and follow-up care. These services include various psychologic, social, and pharmacologic treatments to alleviate symptoms, restore functioning, and prevent relapse of mental disorders. NCCHC further states that the entry screening assessment assists in decisions regarding classification, housing, and the need for mental health services.

Once incarcerated, an inmate should be able to seek mental health and medical care by filling out a Medical Services Request (MSR), a form designed to self-report symptoms and concerns. MSR is a vehicle for care providers to triage the inmate's request to appropriate staff.

The policies and procedures designed to access mental health and medical care must give instructions regarding the assessment process, the imminence of mental health and medical issues and procedures to submit, document, and triage the MSR. The procedure must also identify the medical or mental health staff responsible for addressing the inmate's health concerns.

The policy must address the time to act after receiving an MSR. Inmates with suicidal ideation should be seen by nursing or mental health staff immediately. Inmates with serious mental health symptoms should be seen either by a nurse or mental health professional within twenty-four hours. Inmates with general mental health and psychiatric concerns and requests to visit with a psychiatrist must be seen initially by a mental health professional such as a social worker or a psychologist within seventy-two hours. A psychiatrist's actual visit can be scheduled to take place within fourteen days if the request is for non-emergent reasons. If it is an emergency including active suicidal ideation and behaviors, the psychiatrist visit must be arranged to take place as soon as possible.

A nurse must address requests concerning serious medication side effects and any discrepancies between the ordered and dispensed medications. A nurse may see an inmate with routine mental health issues and then refer him/her to appropriate mental health staff. The inmate may either be seen or be responded to, as clinically indicated, within fourteen days.

Suicide Prevention Policy

The NCCHC Standard[4] states that "each facility identifies suicidal inmates and intervenes appropriately." It further states: "Facility staff identify suicidal inmates and immediately initiate precautions. Suicidal inmates are evaluated promptly by the designated clinician who directs the intervention and ensures follow-up as needed. Acutely suicidal inmates are placed on constant watch. Non-acutely suicidal inmates are monitored on an unpredictable schedule at no more than 15-minute intervals between the checks."

A comprehensive suicide prevention policy that addresses all components is the foundation of a sound suicide prevention program. Key components of a suicide prevention program include the following:

1. Screening/identification
2. Referral

3. Evaluation
4. Housing/monitoring
5. Communication
6. Treatment/intervention
7. Notification
8. Mortality/morbidity review
9. Debriefing
10. Training

SCREENING/IDENTIFICATION

The screening component must specify the tools, methods, and timing of the screening procedure to tackle any potential problems in performing the screening and post-screening procedures.

In most jails and prisons, a mental health professional or a trained correctional officer administers a suicide screening questionnaire (Chapter 3) that captures all known risk factors that predispose and precipitate potential suicidal behavior by an inmate. The screening officer should explore and document all relevant responses. Usually, the screening is done within 24 hours of intake.

A detainee may refuse or be unable to answer questions on the screening instrument due to anger, frustration, personality quirks, intoxication, or florid psychotic symptoms. In this context, the booking officer should ask the detainee to sign a waiver form. If the detainee refuses to sign the waiver, the officer should document his/her refusal and inability to answer questions. If the officer observes any behaviors that lead him or her to believe the detainee may be a threat to themselves or others, the officer should contact the shift supervisor and mental health staff and place the inmate on suicide watch. A proper screening should be conducted as soon as the detainee can cooperate.

While it makes clinical sense to have an adequate suicide screening procedure, courts do not recommend any specific screening form. In *Taylor v. Barkes,*[6] originally filed in 2008, the issue of a particular suicide screening form was raised. Barkes was an inmate with a history of psychiatric and substance use disorders and a prior suicide attempt before he was admitted to a Delaware prison in 2004. Upon admission to the prison, a nurse employed by a medical services contractor performed a suicide screening using a form developed along the model recommended by NCCHC in 1997. It listed seventeen risk factors. The nurse determined that Barkes was not suicidal because he answered only two questions in the affirmative. Therefore, the nurse did not place him under precautions, nor inform a physician of his potential risk. If, according to the jail policy, his responses and nurse's observations indicated that he had at least "eight factors or if certain serious risk factors" were present, she should have notified a physician and placed him on suicide precautions. One evening, during a conversation with his wife, he told her that he would kill himself. His wife did not inform the jail about this conversation and his intent. The next morning the officers found him doing well during regular checks. However, he was found hanging in his cell at noon with a bedsheet.

Barkes's wife and children filed a suit under 42 USC §1983, claiming that the institution violated Barkes's civil rights by failing to prevent his suicide. The suit claimed that Stanley Taylor, the commissioner of corrections, and Raphael Williams, the warden, allegedly violated Barkes's constitutional right to be free from cruel and unusual punishment. However, they were not directly involved in his care. The suit further claimed that they allegedly failed to supervise and monitor the private contractor that performed the intake screening. Taylor and Williams moved for summary judgment on the ground that they were entitled to qualified immunity, but the district court denied the motion, concluding that there were material factual disputes about whether Taylor and Williams had violated Barkes's right by failing to adequately supervise the medical contractor. The court of appeals noted that the medical contractor's suicide screening process did not comply with NCCHC's latest standards, as applicable in 2004, required by the contract.

The U.S. Supreme Court reversed this decision on June 1, 2015, concluding that "No decision of this Court establishes a right to the proper implementation of adequate suicide prevention protocols. No decision of this Court even discusses suicide screening or prevention protocols." The court concluded that the Eighth Amendment does not guarantee access to adequate suicide prevention protocols. Taylor and Williams were granted qualified immunity because in 2004 when Barkes was in prison, no precedent existed that a suicide prevention protocol must be followed.

REFERRAL

A referral to the facility's mental health staff must occur if the initial screening shows that an inmate is at risk or after an officer places an inmate on suicide watch. Failure to refer a potentially suicidal inmate to the shift supervisor and a mental health professional hinders the suicide prevention program's smooth execution. It may form the basis of a future liability claim.

The facility accomplishes the referral on paper, electronically, in person, or through a combination of these. In some systems, a suicide alert is posted electronically on the inmate's record. To avoid "the slip between the cup and the lip," each facility must delineate the referral process, including the medium of referral and any alerts placed on the inmate's record.

EVALUATION

The facility suicide prevention policy must identify the process of suicide risk evaluation, its scope, and the required qualifications of the professional who performs it. The policy must further identify the post-evaluation procedures.

The evaluation must follow a risk assessment protocol that meets the professional standards and state statutory guidelines. A thorough risk assessment must capture the inmate's risk and protective factors (Chapter 3). The determination of risk level (low, medium, or high) directs the appropriate monitoring and treatment. Due to NCCHC's professional standard requiring that only a qualified mental health professional remove an inmate from suicide watch, correctional officers are precluded from this task. The assessment should be completed as soon as possible or within 24 hours.

HOUSING/MONITORING

The assessed risk level determines the type of suicide watch. There are no standardized suicide watch procedures. Though most facilities recognize that a heightened suicide risk level requires some watch, the type of watch and the inmate safety garment requirement during watch vary considerably.

The facility policy must adequately specify the level of risk, type of cell, safety garment requirements, and personal belongings the inmate can keep during suicide watch. The level of observation must be commensurate with the risk level.

Level I: High-Risk—Constant Observation

Inmates at high risk who are acutely or imminently suicidal with an identified plan with intent are classified as high-risk and must receive continuous, uninterrupted observation. The officer who performs the constant observation should have a clear, unobstructed view of the inmate. The officer must document his or her observation at 10-minute intervals. The inmates on constant watch must be placed in an anti-suicide smock, the cell should have only bare minimum personal belongings, and be bereft of anchor points and materials with which inmates could hang themselves.

Level II: Medium Risk—15-Minute Watch

The inmates who are not actively suicidal but express suicidal ideation and plan to commit suicide are classified as medium risk. They must receive 15-minute watch at random, staggered intervals, not exceeding 15 minutes. They are issued an anti- suicide smock and anti-suicide blanket. The cell must be devoid of anchor points and consist of bare minimum personal belongings.

Level III: Low-Risk—Suicide Observation

Level III observation, a step down from Level II, is reserved for inmates with suicidal ideation with no intent or plan. Inmates on this level are issued a jumpsuit or prison uniform, shoes without shoelaces, a mattress, and an anti-suicide blanket. They are placed in a stripped cell, not necessarily a typical suicide observation cell. They should not have any underwear, socks, sheets, sharps, or belts. They are also observed at intervals not to exceed 15 minutes on a staggered basis.

Some facilities use the term psychiatric observation for inmates who warrant close observation due to disturbing and disruptive behaviors. They are observed at intervals not to exceed thirty minutes on a staggered basis. They have all the rights and privileges of an inmate in the general prison/jail population.

POST-SUICIDE WATCH PROCEDURES

The facility post-watch procedure must specify directions regarding mental health service delivery, post-watch follow-up, and the required documentation at every decision point.

A qualified mental health professional who discontinues any watch and step-downs must notify appropriate security staff. In some prisons and jails, the inmate whose level was discontinued receives clinician visits daily for the next three days to ensure the inmate's risk level no longer exists.

COMMUNICATION

Prompt verbal and written communication are important safe-guards for suicide prevention and avoidance of future liability claims. Documentation is the primary form of communication. Prompt recording and reporting of observed behaviors and verbal statements of self-harm by the at-risk inmate must be ensured. Upon completion, the suicide screening form becomes part of the inmate's medical file.

Officers and mental health professionals who observe or become aware of the potentially suicidal behavior of an inmate must promptly document the steps taken. After placing the inmate on watch, the officer should contact the shift supervisor, who then notifies the medical staff or mental health staff. The officer must complete an incident report, which becomes part of the inmate file. All records of inmate monitoring, housing, referrals, and communication by the mental health staff received by the officers must be kept permanently in the inmate's file. Any suicide watch-level change determined by a mental health professional should promptly be recorded in the inmate file.

An observation form is required for inmates on suicide watch. It documents the exact time the inmate is placed in the observation cell, the inmate's observed behavior (sleeping, self-talking, pacing, etc.), and the officer's initials. The form is usually placed on the cell door during the watch, and later becomes part of the inmate file. Officers should observe inmates and document the inmate's behavior as often as determined by the suicide watch level. At shift change, the information regarding suicide watch and observed behaviors should be exchanged with the next officer on duty.

In times of emergency, the officers on site should immediately notify the medical staff, shift supervisor, and facility administrator. They should also be notified any time an inmate is transported to the local emergency room. A physician or the nursing staff should notify the jail or prison's emergency management system. All emergency measures, including CPR and transportation to a local ER, must be documented on incident reports, and made part of the inmate file.

EMERGENCY MANAGEMENT
Another key component is preparedness for emergency management of inmates found hanging. Valuable time will be lost if tools for cutting or loosening the noose are not readily available. In addition, the emergency medical equipment must be in good working order and located in accessible and strategic locations on the housing floor. Officers providing emergency care must wear protective devices when blood and other bodily fluids are present at the location of a medical emergency.

In the case of attempted hanging, lifesaving measures, including CPR, must be initiated as soon as the noose is cut, and the inmate lowered to the floor. While it is important to video record the procedures, time should not be wasted in locating a video camera and chargers.

If medical staff deem it necessary, the inmate will be transported to a local emergency room. A correctional officer must accompany the inmate and observe him at all times in the ER.

The facility administrator will be responsible for determining that each shift has at least one officer with CPR certification.

MORTALITY AND MORBIDITY REVIEW AND DEBRIEFING
Jails and prisons should hold a mortality and morbidity review to analyze the cause and circumstances of inmate deaths or serious injuries. Sometimes, this review is conducted soon after the incident. A more detailed review may be held after a full investigation. The purpose of this review is to determine whether any policy, procedure, or practice has any role in causing or contributing to the suicide or serious injury and institute corrective action. Corrective actions may include the modification of any flawed policies, procedures, and practice.

It may become apparent there is cause to discipline a staff member. Debriefing with the involved officers and mental health professionals should be conducted immediately after the incident.

The Mortality and Morbidity Review team consists of the medical director, mental health director, health services administrator, warden or designee, psychiatrist, and other key personnel.

A sheriff or warden may request an external investigation by a trained investigator, police department, or an investigator from the state department of corrections. Such review and investigation must be conducted objectively. Usually, the investigative report yields valuable information on the causes and circumstances of inmate suicide and serious injuries. The investigative report is usually filed with the facility administrator.

The administrator of the facility must make sure all records, including medical, mental health, and correctional records, any video recording of the emergency lifesaving measures, and the cell are preserved. Sometimes, the site of the incident is declared a "crime scene."

TRAINING

Training of all staff is perhaps the most important tool for suicide prevention. Many lawsuits base their claim of deliberate indifference on inadequate training. The training must offer the officers and the mental health professionals the opportunity to familiarize themselves with the risk factors of inmate suicide, how to identify them, and to take active interventional steps.

The training must focus on three areas:

1. Mental disorders
2. Suicide prevention
3. Policies, procedures, and practice

Mental Disorders:

1. Signs and symptoms of mental disorders
2. Basics of diagnosis of mental disorders per DSM-5
3. Verbal and behavior cues of mentally ill individuals
4. Impact of situational stressors
5. Breakthrough symptoms of mental illness in otherwise stable mentally ill inmates
6. Psychotropic medications and side effects
7. Referral of mentally ill inmates for treatment

Suicide Prevention:

1. The phenomenon of suicide ideation, attempts, and completed suicide
2. Risk and protective factors
3. Methods of suicide
4. Verbal and behavioral cues of self-harm
5. Common myths of suicide
6. Impact of situational stressors and court proceedings
7. Inmate coping skills
8. Suicide risk assessment

Policy, Procedures, and Practice:

1. Screening procedures
2. Suicide watch procedures
3. Housing and cell assignment
4. Classification of detainees/inmates
5. Documentation requirements
6. Communication of detainee/inmate status, screening, and assessment
7. Incident report completion requirements and management
8. Emergency management procedures
9. Use of restraints

Upon initial employment and on an ongoing basis, all correctional and mental health staff should be trained on all aspects of suicide prevention, including mental disorders and suicide prevention policies, procedures, and practices. Mental health professionals rely on their professional skills and training by virtue of their education and license requirements. However, they may still require facility-specific training. Registered nurses and licensed practical nurses must be trained on facility-specific medication administration policies and practices.

The standard practice of initial training consists of four hours of didactic lectures using a syllabus and curriculum covering all areas identified above. Annually, each employee will receive a minimum of two hours of in-service training. Each facility may assign a qualified instructor to provide the training. Initial training is usually provided in a state-run academy. Training modules are included in Appendix I.

TREATMENT

1. *Management of mentally ill inmates*

Retrospective studies show that the mentally ill are over-represented among suicidal inmates,[5] making it pragmatic to establish and manage a mental health services delivery system in each facility. The components of a mental health service delivery system include the following:

    a. Assignment of mental health (MH) score and classification of seriously mentally ill. (MH score assignment is mostly done in the state departments of corrections.)

    b. Administrative segregation management

    c. Crisis management and therapy

    d. Chronic care clinics and regular mental health follow-up

    e. Transfer to inpatient psychiatric care

    f. Tracking of seriously suicidal inmates

The data gathered during the intake, suicide screening, and mental health evaluation helps determine whether an inmate has a serious mental illness. While the correctional officers primarily make the classification and housing assignment, the mental health staff's input is useful when assigning an inmate to a solitary cell or multi-occupancy cell in the general population or a mental health unit (large jails and prisons).

Besides the security and custody scores in prisons, the classification is based on mental health (MH) score assignment, which ranges from 1 to 5. An inmate with no mental health problems may be assigned an MH score of 1. A score of 2 represents mild mental health problems, requiring intervention with the use of medications during a crisis. MH score 3 represents moderate mental health problems with a diagnosed mental disorder. These prisoners are often placed on psychotropic medications. MH score 4 represents severe mental health problems requiring acute management with medications and mental health observation, and MH score 5 represents extreme mental health problems including psychotic symptoms and imminent danger to self or others that often require inpatient psychiatric admission. An inmate who scores 3, 4, or 5 is classified as seriously mentally ill (SMI). Generally, these inmates meet the diagnostic criteria for a psychotic disorder such as schizophrenia and bipolar disorder, major depressive disorder, or severe cognitive impairment. Seriously mentally ill inmates are enrolled in a chronic care clinic where they can be followed with psychotropic medications and supportive therapy. When necessary, acutely mentally ill, and imminently suicidal inmates may be transferred to a state hospital or a crisis stabilization unit, if available within the facility.

Placing a mentally ill inmate in solitary confinement or administrative segregation is counterproductive. The American Psychiatric Association position statement adopted by its board of trustees in 2012 and retained in 2017 states, "Prolonged segregation of adult inmates with serious mental illness, with rare exception, should be avoided due to potential for harm to such inmates. Out of cell therapeutic activities and structured time should be provided."[7] If placed in solitary confinement, some mentally ill inmates decompensate with anxiety, depression, and hopelessness, contributing to suicide propensity. Inmates in administrative segregation must be monitored for suitability of the continued placement, often on a weekly basis with a mental health evaluation and suicide risk assessment by a qualified mental health professional.

In some prisons, crisis stabilization units or crisis management units offer an opportunity to manage the suicidal inmate until the risk is mitigated. Some inmates who engage in multiple suicidal behaviors including attempts and who frequent the crisis stabilization unit require special supervision, medication management, and supportive therapy. While in the crisis stabilization unit, a suicidal inmate is placed on suicide watch until the risk is mitigated.

It is a good practice to track all inmates who have a history of suicide attempts and chronic suicidal ideation. The tracking helps with the early identification of risk and intervention. In some prisons and large jails, an interprofessional committee consisting of clinicians, psychiatrists and administrators, and shift commander monitor the inmates with a suicidal history on a weekly basis.

2. *Psychotropic Medications as a Suicide Prevention Tool*

Proper medication management of mentally ill suicidal inmates is a valuable tool for suicide prevention. Policy and procedures to address the need to prescribe, administer, and monitor psychotropic medications are significant components of a comprehensive suicide prevention program. Before an inmate is placed on medication, an assessment for appropriateness for the use of medications must be completed. The determination may include psychiatric diagnosis, laboratory tests, assessment of clinical risks and benefit, potential drug-to-drug interactions, evaluation of previous medication trials, and assessment of comorbid physical conditions. In addition, previous psychiatric records from the inmate's community health care providers should be obtained and consulted. Inmate consent for treatment should be obtained. Prescriptions and frequency of monitoring must be consistent with clinical standards.

The prescriber should routinely assess and monitor treatment efficacy, adverse reactions, drug interactions, and patient safety. Some psychotropic medications such as mood stabilizers, including lithium, lamotrigine, and valproic acid; and antipsychotic agents such as risperidone, olanzapine, and clozapine may require specific laboratory tests, monitoring, and physical assessments. Long-acting depot form of injectable antipsychotic agents may be prescribed for chronic psychotic patients/inmates.

The use of antipsychotic medications and mood stabilizers requires completion of the Abnormal Involuntary Movement Scale (AIMS) at the initiation of medications as a baseline, when increasing the dose, and every six months.

Laboratory tests such as EKG, blood level of medications, liver function tests, electrolytes, thyroid function tests, complete metabolic panel, complete blood cell count, lipid studies, blood glucose, and HbA1c should be performed as indicated.

All prescriber contacts must be documented with date and time, including the diagnosis, clinical progress, side effects, and rationale for continuation of medications.

Certain procedural safeguards must be in place. It is important to promptly prescribe medications, including "bridging medications," upon admission of an inmate on medications until a physician or psychiatrist evaluates the inmate.

Occasionally, lack of arrangement for bridge medications may be considered a delay in providing appropriate psychiatric care. Those facilities that allow home medications upon admission must process them, employing appropriate safety measures. Those medications may be administered to the inmate with the approval of a physician.

Inter-facility transfer is stressful to mentally ill inmates with suicidal tendencies. Medication must be made available to them upon arrival to the new facility.

A nurse must document all medication and other treatment orders made by a physician immediately upon receiving them. The accuracy and duration of prescriptions and dispensing guidelines in consultation with the pharmacy staff must be ensured. Inmates must receive medications within a reasonable period to avoid undue delay. If there is a non-formulary approval procedure in place, avoid undue delay in the approval and subsequent dispensation.

The dispensing nurse must document on the Medication Administration Record (MAR) that all medications have been administered with the date, time, and inmate refusal. Careful entry of all prescribed medications and any nurse observations on MAR ensures the quality of medication administration. Some inmates refuse medications as a warning before a suicide attempt. A nursing protocol must be in place to intervene in situations where a mentally ill inmate consistently refuses three consecutive doses.

All psychotropic medications must be administered on Direct Observation Therapy (DOT). All medications dispensed to patients on a mental health and suicide watch should be on DOT. DOT is particularly indicated if the prescriber suspects that the inmate/patient may not take the medication as prescribed or is suspected of cheeking the medications.

Some jails allow inmates to keep certain non-psychotropic medication with themselves, known as Keep on Person (KOP) practice. KOP medications must be carefully chosen to avoid those with lethal potential.

3. *Involuntary Medication Administration*

Emergency Use

Psychotropic medication can be administered involuntarily (forced) to an inmate who presents an imminent danger to himself or herself or others due to a severe psychiatric disorder. The forced administration of medication is clinically indicated as a last resort when a mentally ill inmate with a history of a near-lethal suicide attempt makes a serious threat of self-harm with intent and plan. In such a scenario, involuntary medication is likely to immediately reduce imminent danger. The benefits of involuntary medication may outweigh the risks associated with the inmate's incapacity to manage a psychiatric emergency at the time. It may also eliminate the need to transfer to an acute psychiatric unit. Involuntary emergency psychotropic medication such as Haldol can be administered in injectable form in a single dose. (The dose may be determined by the prescribing physician.)

Non-Emergency Use

The U.S. Supreme Court long recognized an inmate's right to refuse treatment based on the Fourteenth Amendment. Such a right must be balanced against the state's right to treat the mentally ill inmate and run a safe institution. Consistent with the Supreme Court decision on *Washington v. Harper*, adequate due process procedures are put in place by many prisons[8] without the requirement of a court review of a medical decision to administer psychotropic medications to a gravely disabled, mentally ill inmate who poses risk to him/herself or others.

Before administering involuntary medications non-emergently, a due process hearing must be held by a treatment review board or committee consisting of a non-treating psychiatrist, a non-treating licensed mental health professional, and an administrator with the psychiatrist as the committee's chair. The committee with the psychiatrist in the majority must decide to administer involuntary medication after careful consideration of all the evidence.

The evidence must include the requirement that the inmate meets the criteria for forced medication. The criteria for non-emergent use of involuntary psychotropic medication should include that the inmate suffers a serious psychiatric disorder consistent with DSM-5 criteria and is gravely disabled, rendering him/her incapable of making treatment decisions and providing for their basic physical needs. Due to impairment in cognitive functioning, reality testing, and volitional control, the inmate should likely do serious harm to themself or others. The prescribed psychotropic medications are likely to reduce suffering, risk, and improve clinical outcomes. In this context, the inmate's refusal to accept pharmacological treatment is a deciding factor to consider involuntary medications.

The committee must provide ample opportunity for the inmate to present evidence and to be represented by a lay advisor. The inmate must have the opportunity to cross-examine any witness and the right to appeal the committee's decision to the designated administrator, who must decide on the appeal within 72 hours.

Often, forced medication approval should be limited to six months. The inmate's need to continue involuntary medication administration must be assessed before the six-month period. Also, the inmate must be provided with the opportunity to accept oral or injectable medication voluntarily at any time during the period.

4. *Detoxification of Alcohol and Substances of Abuse*
Withdrawal from alcohol and opioids is correlated with suicide and serious suicide attempts, more so in jails than prisons. Therefore, all jails should have protocols to assess, detox, and treat alcohol and substance withdrawal. (For details, see Appendix 2)

    a. *Alcohol*

Medication-assisted alcohol detoxification with chlordiazepoxide (Librium) over a period of eight days reduces the withdrawal symptoms and potential medical complications such as delirium tremens, seizures, and suicide vulnerability. Severity assessment of alcohol withdrawal symptoms using a screening instrument such as Prediction of Alcohol Withdrawal Severity Symptoms (PAWSS) must be performed. It is a ten-item questionnaire based on an interview with the inmate concerning his/her history of alcohol intake, intoxication, blackouts, delirium tremens, and other withdrawal symptoms, and clinical evidence of blood alcohol content of >200 mg/dl and the degree of autonomic symptoms such as increased heart rate, tremor, sweating, nausea, and agitation. A score of 4 suggests that the inmate is at risk for a more complicated withdrawal process.

Alcohol withdrawal management that includes use of benzodiazepines falls along one of two models—a scheduled-dosing model or a symptom-driven model. Most jails, even those relatively well-staffed and well-resourced, seldom have the nursing staff for a symptom-driven, or a Clinical Institute Withdrawal Assessment of Alcohol Scale-Revised (CIWA-Ar)-driven approach. Rather, a scheduled-dosing approach is more manageable and just as effective for most patients. In a jail, the treatment regimen[9] can include chlordiazepoxide for 8 days of 25 mg capsule every 6 hours for the first 2 days; followed by 1 capsule every 8 hours for the next 2 days; then 1 capsule every 12 hours for 2 days; and 1 capsule every 24 hours for the final 2 days. The regimen must also include folic acid (vitamin B9) 1 mg daily for 14 days and thiamine (vitamin B1) 100 mg daily for 14 days. If the inmate has a history of complicated alcohol withdrawal that may include seizures, carbamazepine 200 orally 2 times daily for 7 days or Gabapentin 300 orally 3 times daily for 7 days.

b. **Opioids**

Incarceration is a unique opportunity to treat patients for opioid use disorder. Regardless of whether patients are offered a partial agonist, such as buprenorphine, or an antagonist, such as naltrexone, for treatment, all patients withdrawing from opioids should be offered hydration and comfort medications to mitigate withdrawal signs and symptoms. These medications include medications for tremors, diarrhea, nausea/vomiting, and insomnia.

The Food and Drug Administration (FDA) approved buprenorphine/naloxone (Suboxone) for the treatment of opioid use disorders and detoxification. The Drug Addiction Treatment Act of 2000 (DATA 2000) expanded the use of medication-assisted treatment of opioid use disorders by physicians who obtain a waiver to prescribe Suboxone in various treatment settings.

Opiate/heroin withdrawal symptoms can be effectively treated using buprenorphine/naloxone (Suboxone 8/2 mg SL film or tablets). The level of withdrawal symptoms can be assessed using Clinical Opiate Withdrawal Scale (COWS), an eleven-item scale that rates common signs and symptoms of opiate withdrawal and allows them to be monitored over time. The inmate should be in moderate withdrawal before the initial dose of Suboxone is administered.

c. *Benzodiazepines*

Some inmates enter a jail or prison on benzodiazepines such as alprazolam, clonazepam, diazepam, and lorazepam. Commonly, inmates enter the facility on doses significantly higher than the therapeutic doses of these agents. Abrupt discontinuation of high doses of benzodiazepines may precipitate withdrawal symptoms, including agitation, irritability, sleep disturbance, seizures, and acute "rebound anxiety." These symptoms reach their peak between 7 and 14 days. Any potential suicide risk is associated with severe rebound anxiety. Therefore, a protocol to gradually taper benzodiazepines must be initiated to lessen the risk of withdrawal symptoms, rebound anxiety, and potential suicidal risk. Usually, such tapering is done with a 25% reduction of the inmate's entry dose of benzodiazepines every three days over a period of 14 days. During this period, the inmate should be carefully monitored.

VA resources[10] recommend Clonidine 0.1 mg dose twice a day, or Gabapentin 300 mg twice a day or Carbamazepine 400 orally a day during this period. Baclofen or Cyclobenzaprine for muscular cramping for as long as needed may be prescribed.

6. *Use of Restraints*

The use of restraints to protect inmates from self-harm is controversial due to the risk of physical harm this might cause. Restraints may contribute to the death of an inmate in a state of excited delirium,* which occurs more often when (inmate) is restrained in the prone position or with a neck hold.[11]

If used, precautionary measures to prevent inmate injury must be in place. Preferably, the medical director or a psychiatrist must determine if such a restrictive measure can be used. Facilities that use restraints as a suicide prevention procedure must have a policy stating that the facility designates the authority to place and remove the restraints to the shift commander. The restraints should restrict movement only to the degree necessary to prevent self-injury. Inmates on restraints must receive a 15-minute check. Inmates restrained longer than two hours must receive medical attention every two hours. The required medical attention must include postural change, extremities' exercise, and checking medication needs and vital signs. The inmate should be offered food, water, and toilet facilities. Restraints should be removed as soon as the inmate no longer exhibits behavior necessitating restraint. The maximum period the restraints are in place should not exceed 24 hours.

All medical care during restraint should be promptly documented. Additional documentation should include, but not be limited to, the events leading up to the need for restraints, the time the restraints are applied, the justification for their use, observations of the inmate's behavior and condition, 15-minute checks, and the time the restraints were removed.

Despite all these precautionary measures, I strongly discourage the use of restraints as a suicide prevention measure due to the inhumane nature of this procedure and the inherent medical risks.

SUMMARY OF SUICIDE MITIGATION PROGRAM

Suicide prevention strategies can be evaluated only on a retrospective basis. No methodology exists to establish a cause-and-effect relationship between policies, procedures, and practice, and the program's effectiveness (except perhaps a reduction in the number of inmate suicide attempts and suicides during specified periods). I recommend a multidimensional approach with a coordinator to implement the programs. Despite all preventive measures, some inmates provide no clues of their suicidal intent. Then there are those who end their lives accidentally during an apparent attempt.

In summary, the clinical, programmatic, and research-based strategies include the following:

1. Screening of all incoming inmates for suicide risk
2. Comprehensive suicide risk assessment and reassessment at critical points during incarceration
3. Continued risk assessment at every mental health encounter
4. Implementation of legally defensible and clinically sound suicide prevention policies, procedures, and practice
5. Implementation of a comprehensive mental health services delivery system
6. Proper suicide watch procedures when indicated and documentation of watch
7. Tracking all those who are classified as having suicide risk by admitting them to a chronic care clinic
8. Correct classification of the mentally ill inmate and appropriate housing
9. Providing treatment to the seriously mentally ill (SMI) inmates

10. "Watch take" procedure (DOT) for psychotropic medications
11. Medication-assisted treatment of alcohol, opiate, and benzodiazepine withdrawal
12. Medication noncompliance management procedure to capture those inmates who are non-compliant with medications
13. Limit or exclude the prescriptions of benzodiazepines and other medications with abuse potential
14. Timely admission of imminently suicidal inmates to inpatient psychiatric units
15. Involuntary medication administration for those who are gravely disabled but refusing treatment
16. Timely medical intervention for those who are found during suicide attempts
17. Regular staff training to spot and intervene in inmates who are at risk
18. Not placing a mentally ill inmate in solitary confinement
19. Proper administrative segregation management
20. Creating an attitude among the staff that suicides and serious suicide attempts are preventable

CONCLUSION

The multidimensional and multifaceted program involving all stakeholders—administrators, mental health staff, medical staff, and correctional staff—has a greater chance to save lives, restore inmate mental health, and to mount an effective strategy for any potential liability claim.

* Excited delirium is a medical emergency characterized by a sudden onset of symptoms of bizarre and/or aggressive

behavior, shouting, paranoia, panic, violence toward others, unexpected physical strength, and hyperthermia. www.ncbi .nlm.nih.gov. Excited delirium most commonly occurs in males with a history of serious mental illness or acute or chronic substance use disorder, particularly stimulant drugs.

REFERENCES:

1. Woodward v. Correctional Medical Services, 368 F.3d 917 (7th Cir. 2004)

2. Monell v. New York City Dept. of Social Services, 436 U.S. 658 (1978)

3. Daniel, AE. *Preventing suicide in prison: A collaborative responsibility of administrative, custodial, and clinical staff.* Journal of the American Academy of Psychiatry and the Law 34(2) (2006) 165–175

4. NCCHC standards for mental health services in correctional facilities (2018)

5. Daniel, AE and Fleming, J. *Suicides in a State Correctional System 1992–2002:* A Review. Journal of Correctional Health Care 12 [(1) (2006) 24–35

6. Taylor v. Barkes, 135 S. Ct 2042 2015

7. *American Psychiatric Association Position Statement on Segregation of Prisoners with Mental Illness, approved by the Board of Trustees, December 2012 and retained in December 2017.* www.Psychiatry.org

8. Washington v. Harper, 494 U.S. 210 (1990)

9. Rottnek, F, and Menzies,P. *ARCA Medicine Guidelines* (2020)

10. https://www.va.gov/PAINMANAGEMENT/docs/OSI_1 _Toolkit_Pain_Educational_Guide.pdf

11. Pollanen, MS, Chiasson, DA, Cairn, JT and Young, JG, *Unexpected death related to restraint for excited delirium: a retrospective study of deaths in police custody and in the community* CMAJ 158 (12) 1603–1607

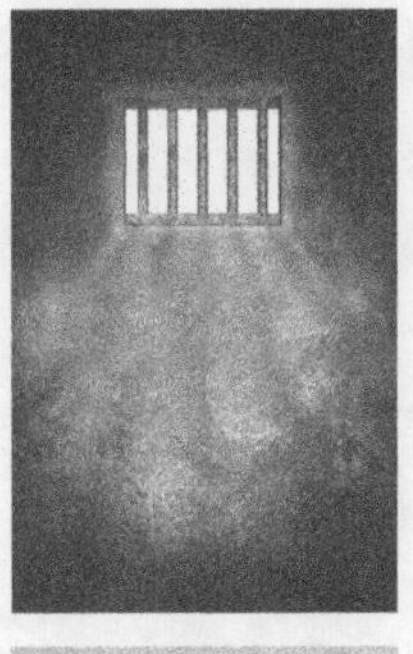

CHAPTER 5

BEST PRACTICES BY CORRECTIONAL STAFF

Lt. Richard Lichten (Ret.), Jail and Police Policies and Procedures expert

Richard Lichten (Lt. Ret.) is an expert consultant on police and jail procedures for attorneys, public agencies, and the media. His areas of expertise include Use of Force, TASER, Police Practices, Narcotics, and Jail and Prison/Custody practices, including experience and training in jail medical care policy, jail suicide prevention, and jail suicide risk management. Mr. Lichten holds an instructor certification in suicide prevention and in risk management in patrol and in jails. He also holds certification as an Arrest-Related and In-Custody Death Investigative Specialist by the Institute for the Prevention of In-Custody Deaths (IPICD). He has provided expert testimony in state and federal courts throughout the United States in police and jail procedures. www. PoliceandJailProcedures.com

The best practices by correctional staff to prevent suicides relate to:

1. inmate safety;
2. safety of correctional staff; and
3. procedures and practice designed to avoid liability claims.

All correctional staff must be integrally involved in inmate suicide prevention and inmate management. Each facility must function like a well-oiled machine to meet the correctional system's goals of retribution, deterrence, and rehabilitation while maintaining inmate safety.

Once an arrestee has been accepted into a jail or prison, he or she becomes an inmate whose basic human needs and supervision rests with the correctional facility and staff. Regardless of the official title, the correctional officer for all intent and purposes functions as both an inmate caretaker and risk manager.

While several national organizations, such as the American Correctional Association (ACA) and the NCCHC, provide institutional and health-care-focused accreditation, many U.S. jails and prisons are not accredited. However, all states and municipalities have some inmate supervision and management standards in place.

This chapter presents the basics that facilities should have in place to optimize inmate well-being while mitigating inmate suicide risk. The title "correctional officer" is used when describing the duties and responsibilities of deputy sheriffs, custody assistants/technicians, jail or prison officers, or police officers responsible for overseeing the safety of inmates. The term "reasonable correctional officer" refers to a typical correctional officer with basic officer training, and who, in a comparable situation, will respond similarly. A reasonable correctional officer is trained to know that if the best practices are not followed properly, and an inmate harms him or herself, the officer may be held accountable and/or legally liable, both personally and as a representative of the facility.

NO WORDS NEED BE SPOKEN

An inmate needs to report that he/she is suicidal to obligate action on the part of a correctional officer. Correctional officers must monitor the inmate's behaviors that are consistent with known facts about inmate suicidal ideation and behaviors. Suppose a trained correctional officer sees a crying inmate standing in a cell holding a jail-made knife (shank) to his/her throat. In that case, the officer does not have to hear the inmate say, "I am suicidal" to form a reasonable belief that the inmate poses a danger to him/herself.

It is not unusual for suicidal inmates to deny their suicide ideation. Most inmates know if they admit to suicide ideation, they will be stripped of clothes, given suicide protective garments, locked down in a more restrictive environment, and closely watched. If an inmate wishes to harm him/herself, it is much easier to deny suicidal thoughts or say nothing.

TYPE OF FACILITIES

In the United States, several types of custody facilities are designed to hold inmates. The most common custody facilities include the following:

1. Detention centers
2. Lockups
   a. Police station lockups
   b. Courthouse lockups
   c. Jails
   d. Prisons
      - State
      - Federal

DETENTION CENTERS

The term *detention center* refers to a facility where detainees/ inmates—especially those awaiting processing, trial, sentencing, or extradition—are held in custody for short periods. Examples of detention centers include juvenile detention centers, immigration and customs enforcement detention centers, and family staging centers.[1]

LOCKUPS

Most local police and sheriff patrol stations have a lockup wherein arrestees are held until being transported to the county jail, usually in a day or two.

If inmates are in custody while attending a trial, they will be kept in courthouse lockups during trial days and return to jail after their trial concludes. Depending on where the jail or courthouse is located, inmates may be awakened for breakfast and transported to the courthouse as early as 4:00 a.m. and may return to their jail cells as late at 10:00 p.m.

City and county jails hold inmates pending trial, during the trial, and awaiting sentencing and transportation to a state or federal prison. Inmates who receive a sentence of less than a year often serve their sentence in jails.

Types of jails: Some jails are considered temporary; they hold persons for only a few days (station lockups). Some hold both pretrial detainees and sentenced inmates, while others hold only the sentenced. Some jails hold inmates who are court-ordered to work-release programs. One or more of these jails may be housed in a building or jail complex. Jail capacity may range from a handful of inmates to thousands.

Once inmates have been sentenced, they may be sent to a state or federal prison, based on their charges and their court venue. Prisons are typically divided into minimum-, medium-, and maximum-security facilities. Since prisons are typically run by states or by the Federal Bureau of Prisons, there tends to be more consistency in prison administration and policy than in jails.

Jails and prisons house inmates in single-occupancy or multi-occupancy cells, or dormitory-style housing units with single beds or bunk beds.

ROLES AND RESPONSIBILITIES OF FACILITY PERSONNEL

Administrators:
All facilities are overseen by administrators who ensure its overall safety and operation. The administration of a jail rests with the sheriff, and that of a prison with the chief administrator. Administrators contract with private vendors, large and small, to provide mental health, medical, dental, pharmacy, commissary, and other services. In addition to maintaining the facility's

overall safety and the security of the inmates, administrators are responsible for developing and implementing the following:

1. Policies and procedures for inmate health care
2. Providing or securing necessary inmate medical and mental health treatment
3. Policies and procedures of suicide prevention and intervention
4. Policies and procedures relating to the control, delivery, and administration of prescription and nonprescription medications
5. Policies and procedures relating to the provision of inmate programs and services
6. Employee training policies, procedures, and practice, and adherence to relevant laws, rules, regulations, standards, and prison policies

Captains command a facility's functions and operations and are held accountable for inmate safety. They ensure the correctional staff receives up-to-date, ongoing, detailed training on inmate suicide prevention.

Lieutenants are responsible for a shift at a facility. Typically, there are three shifts: graveyard/early morning shift, day shift, and afternoon shift. Lieutenants manage the operations of their assigned shift and ensure that the sergeants and correctional officers follow policies and procedures, including that of suicide prevention. Lieutenants do not develop procedures that cover all shifts; that is the role of captains.

Sergeants supervise correctional officers. They ensure that the correctional officers follow policies and procedures. Sergeants are usually considered first-line supervisors.

Correctional officers are responsible for the direct supervision of inmates. They ensure inmates follow facility rules. Perhaps one of the most important jobs of a correctional officer is to ensure that inmates under their care do not engage in criminality or prohibited behaviors (e.g., fighting, escape, sharing/selling medications), and are not in medical distress.

PROCESSING AN ARRESTEE

Correctional officers are the eyes and ears of the suicide prevention program—from an inmate's arrival to their release from the facility. The officers' key overall role is to ensure the inmates and mental health staff's safety and security. They also escort inmates to medical, mental health, and psychiatric appointments.

At the time of arrest, an arrestee may appear depressed and show erratic behaviors that raise suspicion that he or she may be potentially dangerous to him/herself. Occasionally, an arrestee may verbalize suicidal thoughts.

Sometimes, the arresting officer may decide to transport the arrestee to a local hospital for medical clearance or to commit an arrestee to a local psychiatric hospital, depending on the arrestee's medical, emotional, and behavioral status.

In processing an arrestee who makes a suicidal statement or is suspected of having suicidal tendencies, the arresting officer must take the following steps:

1. Thoroughly search the arrestee and take away all their personal property, especially shoes with laces and other items that can be used for self-injury.

2. Verbally inform the jail's intake staff that the arrestee has expressed suicidal ideation or has threatened suicide.
3. Document the name of the correctional officer who has been informed of the arrestee's suicidal ideation.
4. Complete the standard booking forms, which should include the suicidal ideation information.

Once the arresting officer has handed over the arrestee's property and completed the booking process and the arrestee has been accepted into the custody of the receiving facility, the arresting officer's responsibility to the arrestee ends. The arrestee is now considered an inmate and is the responsibility of the correctional staff.

The correctional officer at the receiving facility performs the following:

1. Assigns a booking number for the inmate
2. Completes the medical and mental health intake questionnaires, which are normally a part of the booking process. These forms are sometimes called intake screening forms. The correctional officer asks the inmate about his/her suicide threat made to the arresting officer. The officer makes certain to address all the questions on the mental health intake screening form. If the newly arrived inmate denies being suicidal, the officer should consider the inmate to be suicidal until a mental health provider evaluates him or her. In smaller facilities, there are no medical or mental health providers at the jail during the time of arrival of the arrestee.

3. Assigns inmate housing, usually in the general population, if warranted. If the inmate is determined to be suicidal, he/she will be placed in a suicide observation cell under suicide watch, per the facility's protocol.
4. Informs the medical and mental health staff of the inmate's placement under suicide watch and the inmate's threat of suicide
5. Documents the same on paper and/or electronic record

OFFICERS' SUPPORTIVE ROLE IN INMATE MENTAL HEALTH CARE

For the delivery of mental health care to inmates, correctional officers play a supportive role by assisting with escorting the inmate to mental health appointments. If correctional staff fails to bring the inmate to mental health appointments, the necessary inmate care may be delayed.

An officer can provide valuable information regarding inmates' mental health status and changes. For instance, the officer can observe and report to the mental health staff an inmate's sudden mental status changes, withdrawal from peers, refusal to eat and drink, crying spells, giving away possessions, and isolative and erratic behaviors such as smearing feces on surfaces, psychotic behaviors, and behaviors that may result from medication side effects.

Like mental health clinicians, correctional officers may observe specific changes in potentially suicidal inmates during days or weeks before the attempt. Behavioral changes such as withdrawal from staff and other inmates, seeking privacy by insisting on being transferred to a single- or a double-person cell, seeking excessive medications, refusing medications or food, and refusing to take showers are common. Some request earlier appointments with a therapist or a psychiatrist. Repeat medical service requests are another indicator.

Along with these behavior changes, some emotional signs and symptoms are worth noting. Preceding the suicide act, the inmate may exhibit extreme anger, severe agitation, or mood changes. Some may entirely withdraw from interaction after making the final decision. Some may make direct or oblique statements to fellow inmates. Some may inquire if euthanasia is an option.

Correctional officers must take inmates' suicidal thoughts, threats, or behaviors seriously; they must not question the legitimacy of such thoughts or actions. At no time should an officer claim that an inmate is joking about suicide statements. If there are any actions, words, or utterances which lead an officer to believe that an inmate may be thinking of suicide, the officer should take all steps necessary to ensure the inmate's safety.

In cases of apparently feigned gestures (superficial marks, hesitation marks, an injury that is not life-threatening, or the inmate has not displayed any wish to commit suicide), the inmate must still be examined by the medical/mental health professional and have the examination documented. Inmates can accidentally kill themselves in an act intended to be a gesture.

In facilities where officers are tasked with dispensing medications to inmates, officers must make sure inmates swallow the medicines under their direct observation. To allow an inmate to walk away with pills in his/her hand is to invite that inmate to hoard medications, which may be used to overdose later.

If an inmate wishes to refuse medication, such refusal must be face-to-face with the nursing staff. It is outside an officer's scope of the responsibility to accept an inmate's refusal of medication. If the inmate refuses to exit the cell to make the refusal to the nursing staff, the nurse must go to the inmate and take his refusal at his cell.

INMATE SAFETY CHECK

Most U.S. jails and prisons require routine inmate safety checks, as per institutional policy and state regulations. Inmate safety checks may be required hourly or several times an hour, depending on the needs of the inmates and the facility. The safety checks should not be confused with the required inmate counts conducted to ensure each inmate assigned to the jail or prison is accounted for and has not escaped.

Conducting proper inmate safety checks is one of the most important duties a correctional officer performs during his/her shift. In a dormitory setting, the officer must enter the dorm and get close enough to conduct direct visual observation of inmates. It is not a proper safety check if the officer stands at the entrance and glances at the dorm. Supervisors may also perform safety checks, known as incidental checks, by looking into the dormitories and cells as they walk around the facility.

Safety checks are also required in administrative segregation and disciplinary housing areas. Inmates in disciplinary housing often have a higher degree of depression and suicidal ideation than inmates housed in the general population. For this reason, it is critical to perform safety checks every thirty minutes or more often. When observing inmates in the disciplinary housing (and anywhere in the jail), at the first hint of an inmate suffering a mental health crisis, no matter how seemingly minor, he/she should be referred immediately to medical/mental health professionals.

Inmate safety checks ensure that the inmates:

1. are not involved in criminal or prohibited behaviors such as gambling, making weapons, drug usage, and fighting;
2. are not experiencing trauma caused by other inmates;
3. are not in the process of attempting suicide or other self-injurious behaviors; and
4. are not in any acute medical distress, (e.g., shortness of breath, chest pain, and choking).

UNOBSTRUCTED VIEWS

Officers should have a direct view of the inmate under suicide watch and inmate safety check. Therefore, no obstruction to the cell view must be permitted.

Sometimes, due to the cells' layouts, there may be a privacy wall next to the toilet. If the privacy wall hinders an officer's direct visual observation, he/she should instruct the inmate to move into view. If the officer cannot get the inmate to respond to his/her command, the officer will summon backup and enter the cell to check on the inmate.

The direct view is obstructed when an inmate covers up the cell window or uses a blanket to cover his or her head while sleeping—not an uncommon occurrence. Besides not being able to see if there is an actual inmate under the blanket, the officer cannot discern whether the inmate is breathing or suffering medical distress.

Officers must instruct inmates not to fully cover up with their blankets. Should they do so and fall asleep, they should be awakened so their health status can be assessed by direct visual observation. Of course, inmates should not be needlessly disturbed or aroused. Nevertheless, to properly conduct inmate safety checks, officers must insist that inmates show themselves for the safety check.

Should an inmate not respond to the officer's commands, in addition to getting backup to go inside the cell, the officer should, in an abundance of caution, call for the nurse to respond to the situation.

SUICIDE WATCH

Failure to conduct proper suicide watch is a significant causal factor in many attempted and completed suicides. An assigned correctional officer provides a regular visual check of the inmate on suicide watch at least every 15 minutes on a staggered basis. During these checks, the officer converses with the inmate, if possible. The check is documented each time with the time/date, name of the officer who checked, and the inmate's behaviors, such as sleeping, standing, eating, or any abnormal status. These logs are placed in the inmate's file.

A suicide observation cell is a specially designated cell, thoroughly searched for any potential anchors for hanging. The suicidal inmate is issued a suicide-resistant smock and a blanket made of heavy cloth that is nearly impossible to tear.

The correctional officer also ensures the cell's intercom system works properly for the inmate to call for help in an emergency.

TIME REQUIRED FOR A PROPER SAFETY CHECK

Much more than a passing glance is required to conduct a proper safety check. If, during a safety check, the correctional officer walks by and glances at an inmate who, for example, may be sitting at a desk reading, the officer would know the inmate is alive but would not know if the inmate suffers from medical distress. If the inmate is in his/her bunk and appears to be sleeping, flashing a light into a darkened cell window for a second to locate the inmate inside the cell is not a proper safety check. The officer must get close enough to see each inmate and look long enough to determine if the inmate is not in medical distress or involved in any prohibited behaviors.

The average adult has a respiration rate between 12 to 20 times a minute. It would take at least three seconds to watch an intake of breath if the person's breathing rate was 20 times a minute. If the person is breathing at a slower rate of 12 times a minute, it will take at least five seconds to see the person take a breath. To reiterate, a passing glance is not a proper safety check.[1]

Problems associated with a safety check and logging are highlighted in the following example. Should the inmate safety log show that an officer conducted an official safety check of 145 sleeping inmates in under three minutes—that's evidence of an *improper* safety check. It is physically impossible to view each inmate long enough to see if they are breathing, let alone suffering medical distress, during this limited time. If the officer spends a minimum of three seconds per inmate to see if they take at least one breath, at a rate of 20 times a minute, it will take 7.5 minutes to view each inmate effectively. If all 145 inmates breathe at the slower rate of 14 times a minute, then 9.6 minutes would be needed to view each sleeping inmate properly. That time does not include the time it takes to walk around the living area, go up and down the stairs if needed, and check on inmates who may be fully covered.

In the example above, since there is no way a proper safety check of 145 inmates could be done in under three minutes, then not only did this safety check not benefit the inmate, but also the officer falsified the log, an official document.

VIDEO MONITORS

Many jails and prisons use video monitors to supervise inmates and for overall security. The use of video monitors should never replace actual eyes-on monitoring, especially for suicidal inmates.

The Institute for the Prevention of In-Custody Deaths (IPICD) warns that video monitors are not a replacement for in-person, eye-on safety inmate checks. Correctional officers must be close enough to see skin and ensure the inmate is breathing. A proper safety check is done by direct visual observation, not by video.[2]

If video monitors are used, certain safeguards must be in place:

1. Monitor is used to supplement the visual check
2. One person must actively watch the monitors.

3. Limit the number of videos monitored at the same time.
4. Determine who audits the recordings.
5. Determine the time frame for storage and retrieval of the videos
6. The facility administrator must promptly address any unusual activities noted on the monitors.

An officer in a control booth who is multitasking, answering the telephones, opening cell doors, watching inmates in the common areas, and keeping logs cannot be expected to actively watch a video monitor.

SAFETY CHECK LOG AND LOGBOOKS

When safety checks are conducted, the officer conducting the check must log the time of the check and his/her observations of the inmate at the time of the check. Whatever the officer observes the inmate doing at the time of the check must be accurately reflected in the safety check log. Also, the written logs must correspond with the video checks.

During a shift, a supervisor must observe staff performing safety checks and verify the accuracy of the logs. The supervisor must inspect and sign the logbooks once a shift. This inspection should not be done at the start of the shift. If the logbook concerns a linear row of cells, it should be kept at the very end of the row. The officer doing the check must walk to the end to write in the book. One way for the supervisor to ensure the accuracy of safety checks is to inspect the logbooks every shift.

The old dictum, "If it isn't documented, it didn't happen," is apt here. When an attempted or completed suicide is discovered, the supervisor should control the concerned logbooks and log sheets because they would become evidence in a potential lawsuit. This way, the administration can defend against allegations of log tampering after the fact.

Training must focus on the possibility that attempted and completed suicides often occur right after the safety checks are completed. If the safety checks are not done properly and accurately, if needed, emergency medical care of the inmates would be delayed.

PROCEDURES WHEN AN INMATE IS FOUND HANGING
When an inmate is found hanging, correctional officers and supervisors each play an important role in saving the inmate's life.

It is not uncommon for other inmates to sound the alarm of "man down" when they see an inmate hanging. A correctional officer may discover the hanging inmate during a safety check or just walking by during what is called an incidental safety check. Once an inmate is found hanging, a correctional officer should immediately summon help, including medical care and fire department paramedics. While waiting for help, any other inmates who are nearby should be locked down at once.

It is difficult for a lone correctional officer to lift a hanging inmate. Usually, two officers are required to lift the inmate up while a third officer uses a cut-down tool to cut the ligature. Once the inmate is lowered to the floor, correctional officers, and medical staff (if available), would provide lifesaving treatment, including CPR, until relieved by emergency medical personnel.

Officers who discover inmates in cardiac arrest or not breathing, from hanging or other reasons, should not wait for the medical staff to start lifesaving measures, including CPR, due to the urgency of the situation. Delay in initiating lifesaving measures puts the inmate in further peril. It could also be considered as evidence for a potential deliberate indifference claim.

If medical personnel decide to transfer the inmate to a local hospital, a correctional officer accompanies the inmate to the hospital and stays with him or her until relieved of duty.

The inmate's cell is considered a crime scene, so supervisors must ensure it is cordoned off. They must also secure housing area logbooks, which are considered evidence. Any video of the cell and the activities related to the lifesaving measures must be secured. Supervisors should have the other inmates in the area interviewed as witnesses. All involved corrections personnel should write thorough incident reports consistent with the facility policy.

Once suicide is discovered, the area needs to be locked down as if a homicide had occurred. No one enters the crime scene after the inmate is removed or pronounced dead. Should the inmate be pronounced dead, the body should not be touched.

Start a crime scene log and tape off the area. Look for witnesses. If witnesses are found, separate them. Identify and fully question persons who were able to see what happened—even if they say they saw nothing. Do not look for physical evidence until told to do so by the investigators. Do not contaminate the scene. Await directions from homicide detectives.

DEBRIEFING

A debriefing is a required procedure after a critical event such as a completed suicide or a serious suicide attempt. A debriefing is not an investigation. The debriefing brings together the involved personnel for an open and honest discussion of the situation and circumstances of the incident to gain insight and understanding of what occurred and improve responses for a future critical incident. The debriefings should always include candid discussions about what went right, what went wrong, and lessons learned.

The involved personnel are brought together soon after the event. The following procedure is recommended for the debriefing meeting:

1. The supervisor who functions as the incident commander leads the debriefing.
2. On a chalkboard or whiteboard, the supervisor writes What went right?" and "What went wrong?" in two columns.
3. Then, going around the room, everyone gets a chance to report what went right in one or two words. For example, if the medical response was good, then the words might be "medical response." If the radio communication went well, the words might be "radio communication." All the words are then listed on the board.
4. Then, going around the room, everyone gets a chance to report what went wrong in one or two words. For example, if keys to a gate/door failed to work, the words might be "bad keys," or if the suicide response kit did not have a cut-down tool, the words might be "no cut-down tool." All the words are then listed on the board.

5. A discussion follows. "Lessons learned" is written on the board, and an open discussion takes place.
6. Finally, a list of recommendations to improve handling of a future critical incident is developed.
7. The supervisor will write a report of the meeting procedures and recommendation and forward it to the jail administrator.

INVESTIGATION

Facility administrators conduct a thorough, objective, and impartial investigation to determine if policies and procedures were followed. It is important to begin the investigation soon after the critical incident. Failure to investigate a critical incident such as a suicide attempt or completed suicide thoroughly and quickly may show an effort by the facility to ignore or bend the evidence to a predetermined conclusion that the facility personnel followed proper policies and procedures.

USE OF FORCE

Police and correctional officers may find it necessary to use force against mentally ill persons with suicidal behaviors. This force can range from a simple touch on arm to "control holds," use of pepper spray, baton, or taser, to the use of deadly force.

Statistics from the U.S. Bureau of Justice show that there are eighteen thousand federal, state, county, and local law enforcement agencies,[3] each with its own definition of "use of force." The use of force may be best defined as an intentional act by an officer who knows or should know that it may cause pain or injury to a subject for the lawful purpose of controlling his or her actions. The primary objective for using force is to gain or regain control of an out-of-control person or situation. There are two kinds of force: spontaneous use of force, when, without warning, an officer is attacked, and planned use of force, such as when an armed mentally ill person is in a home threatening a family member. Another example of a planned use of force is a jail inmate who is suicidal and threatening to hang himself or herself and refusing to comply with correctional officers' orders.

Officers must use de-escalation tactics, safety permitting, whenever possible before resorting to force. Sometimes, there is no time to de-escalate, especially when spontaneous use of force is required to stop the threat. De-escalation methods include actions by officers to avoid using force unless immediately needed to protect someone or stop dangerous actions. Of course, once the risk of danger has passed, the officer should not use further force. Any further use of force may be considered excessive force.

Proven methods to de-escalate, time and safety permitting, include, but are not limited to:

1. giving orders to the subject/inmate slowly;
2. allowing the person receiving the orders time to fully understand what is being ordered, especially when dealing with known mentally ill or suicidal person who may have difficulty processing orders and commands;
3. allowing the person additional time to comply with orders before force is used; and
4. slowing down the tempo of the situation, considering time, distance, and communication style.

Officers need to consider the possibility that the person may be non-compliant due to a medical condition. These may include physical or hearing impairment, seizures, drug effects, diabetic emergencies, and/or a state of excited delirium, and may, therefore, require a medical response. Language barrier must also be considered in dealing with the situation. Time permitting, officers should consider the use of crisis negotiators and/or specially trained mental health response teams. If possible, uninvolved inmates should be removed from the area to lower the stress of the involved inmate.

SAFETY MEASURES, CHECKS, AND AUDITS

Cell design

Cells need to be free of anything that can be used as an anchor to tie off a noose. To achieve this, hang-resistant cells may be designed to eliminate all potential anchors, for example, towel hooks. The sink should have curved spigots so a cord/rope will slide off them. Water handles should be designed so they cannot be used as an anchor. Air vent grates must be small, so an inmate cannot snake a torn sheet through them. If the bunk is welded to the wall, care should be taken to eliminate the gap between the wall and the side of the bunk.

Telephone cords

All telephone cords shall be at a length that prevents its potential use as a ligature: Even if the length of the cord is the shortest possible to retain functionality, it is still possible for an inmate to hang himself. It is advisable to avoid a corded phone in lock up detention cells. In one case the suicidal inmate used his pants as the noose and tied one leg of the pant to the short telephone cord.

Window coverings

The primary purpose of a cell window is to see the inmate inside the cell. It makes no sense to have a window covering on the outside of the cell window as it prevents safety checks.

Never allow inmates to cover up their cell windows from inside. Experience has shown that this is a warning sign of an inmate suicide attempt. If a window is found covered, take steps to remove it as quickly as possible.

Cell searches and inspections

Regular—although varied in time—and spontaneous cell searches should be done and the searches should be documented in the appropriate logbooks. Supervisors need to inspect and sign off on these logbooks once a shift. Regularly, cells used for suicide watch need to be thoroughly searched for contraband and inspected for defects such as tie-off points (towel hooks) and needed repairs, such as air vent grates. Each time the cell is searched and inspected, be sure to document who conducted the search or inspected the cell and document any needed repairs.

In-house roll call/briefings

Routine distribution of bulletins on suicide prevention is good practice. Document when the bulletins are handed out and when suicide prevention is discussed at roll call/briefings.

Ensuring proper response by medical staff
In a medical/mental health emergency, supervisors must ensure that sufficient medical personnel respond as needed. There have been cases where only one nurse responded, and other nurses opted to remain away and not assist in the emergency.

Use of video recordings with audio
When dealing with an inmate with suicidal tendencies, physical interactions between the inmate and custody staff should be videotaped as much as possible. For example, if an inmate who has been violent in the past is to be removed from his/her cell and taken to an interview, the entire move should be videotaped. It is important to start the video before the cell door is opened. If the video starts after the cell door is opened and there is a need for force, and it was not captured on video, allegations of staff misconduct would be difficult to defend. The camera should stay on until the inmate is returned to his/her cell. The videotape should then be dated and stored. In all videotaped cases, a supervisor must be present for the duration of the taping.

Taking photographs or video recording of attempted suicides or completed suicides for staff's personal use must be strictly prohibited.

Suicide intervention kits
Each facility must make sure that suicide intervention kits containing a cut-down tool, rubber gloves, towel, and large trauma bandages are well placed throughout the jail. Supervisors must ensure that officers inspect the kits each shift and that the inspection is documented.

Nursing supervisors must make sure that nurses inspect emergency medical equipment (oxygen tanks, for example) at the start of each shift and document that the inspection was done.

Suicide response drills

Each facility must hold periodic, regular, verifiable (documented) suicide response drills. The drills, under the direction of supervisors, should include:

1. randomly questioning the staff about policies and procedures on suicide prevention;
2. inspection of suicide intervention kits;
3. staff's response to a hanging, wrist cutting, overdosing, and verbal threat; and
4. lifesaving measures including CPR with a CPR mannequin.

SUICIDE PREVENTION PROGRAM AUDIT

The correctional components of the facility's suicide prevention program should be audited annually to determine whether the correctional staff complied with the suicide prevention policies, procedures, and practice and as a quality assurance tool. The audit must preferably be conducted by an experienced auditor not associated with the facility. Such audits may be ordered by the sheriff of a jail or a prison warden.

The audit should cover the following:

1. Processing of an arrestee
2. Screening protocol by the officers
3. Accuracy of classification and housing of inmates
4. Compliance with safety and suicide watch procedures

5. Use of safety garments
6. Onsite review of two to three inmates on suicide watch
7. Accuracy of safety logs
8. Critical incident procedures including protocol after the incident
9. Documentation and processing of medications brought in by the detainee or by family members
10. Testing and training of processes for medication administration—if the facility assigns the task to officers
11. Documentation of communication from family members and concerned people
12. Training schedules and lesson plans, and officer participation and personnel file entries of the training
13. Audit findings and conclusions transmitted to the sheriff and warden should be used to determine if any change in procedures and practices are warranted

COMMON LIABILITY LAWSUITS INVOLVING OFFICERS

The following vignettes illustrate common scenarios found in liability claims against correctional officers.

1. An inmate hanged himself in his cell. While performing a scheduled safety check, the officer was seen on the video staring at his cell phone and failing to look through cell window as he walked by the hanging inmate.
2. An officer thought an inmate lying on his bunk totally covered with a blanket was sleeping. The officer did not take steps to ensure the inmate was alive and not in medical distress. This inmate had been dead for hours.

3. An inmate in a darkened cell, with a history of attempted suicide, had chewed a "hole" on his arm, causing severe bleeding. The officers who conducted the safety checks only glanced into the darkened cell for less than a second. The inmate was found dead hours later.

4. An inmate with a history of mental illness, housed in a crisis stabilization unit, gouged out his eyes during a 30-minute period. The safety checks were late by 30 minutes. Had the checks been done on time, emergency medical care could have been summoned much sooner.

5. An inmate was booked into a jail with active symptoms of methamphetamine intoxication. He was held in a cell. The safety checks were logged on time, but the video showed the correctional officers walking up to the cell and glancing into the cell for less than a second while the inmate lay on the floor in acute medical distress. The inmate died an hour or so after booking.

6. An inmate made his suicide ideation known during booking. He was placed alone in a holding cell pending transport to a medical unit a few miles away. He was not checked on for hours. He used one leg of his pants to make a noose, tied the other leg to the exposed telephone cord, and hanged himself.

7. Family members of an inmate called the jail and informed the staff of the inmate's suicide intent. No action was taken by the correctional officers who took these calls. The inmate successfully committed suicide a short time later.

8. A correctional officer saw a braided rope made from a bedsheet hanging from the cell's light fixture but took

no action. The next day the required cell safety checks were not performed properly. The inmate was found hanging from this braided rope.

9. An inmate who expressed suicidal ideation was improperly classified to an administrative segregation unit instead of a high observation medical/mental health unit for suicide watch. Once the inmate was placed into the administrative segregation (Ad Seg) unit, he was issued a bedsheet. This was against policy. The inmate used the bedsheet to hang himself.

10. Using the cell's intercom, an inmate asked about euthanasia for inmates serving long prison sentences. The officer told the inmate euthanasia was not an option. The inmate replied that he was serious about this. The officer followed the existing policy and informed the housing staff. That inmate hanged himself in between the hourly safety checks.

REFERENCES:

1. https://www.ice.gov/detain/detention-management

2. Prevention of In-Custody Deaths (IPICD) and from California POST (Peace Officer Standards in Training) basic first aid training

3. https://www.bjs.gov/content/pub/pdf/nsleed.pdf

PART II

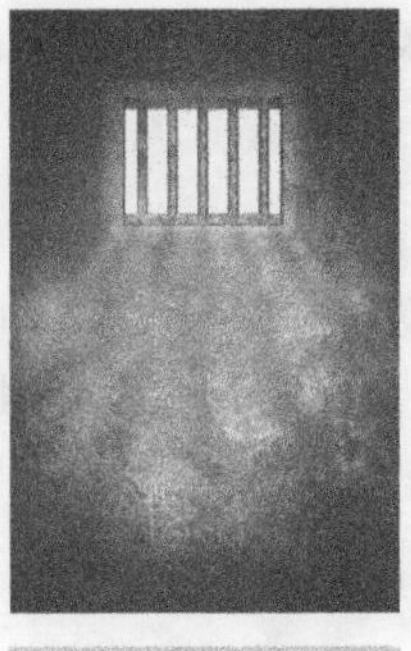

CHAPTER 6

LITIGATION RELATED TO SUICIDE AND SUICIDE ATTEMPTS

I have included this chapter to give expert consultants a general overview of issues they may encounter analyzing, consulting, and testifying on cases involving suicide in jails and prisons. Acknowledging that I am not a lawyer or an expert legal analyst, I have become, nonetheless, aware of commonly litigated issues based on expert analysis and consultation on seventy-five cases in various jurisdictions in the U.S.

Correctional experts must know the nature of litigation, pertinent standards of proof, underlying legal principles in decision-making, and a few landmark cases related to suicide in jails and prisons. Historically, case law related to deliberate indifference-based claims evolved beginning in the mid-1970s by acknowledging the prisoner's constitutional right to adequate health care.

Suicide and serious suicide attempts by inmates can cause several types of legal claims:

1. Medical negligence
2. Negligence by correctional staff
3. Deliberate indifference
4. Americans with Disabilities Act (ADA) claims

Medical malpractice is based on state law, and §1983 actions (deliberate indifference) are based on federal law. Both types of claims can be brought in either state or federal courts, but §1983 cases are removable to federal court because they arise under federal law. Sometimes, malpractice and deliberate indifference claims may be made simultaneously. Negligence claims against the correctional staff arise under state law and are generally litigated in state courts. ADA claims related to suicide commonly accompany deliberate indifference claims.

Legal issues including qualified immunity and deliberate indifference are interpreted differently by different courts. Likewise, legal principles supporting a medical malpractice claim vary from state to state.

MEDICAL NEGLIGENCE (MALPRACTICE)

Nature of the claim

A medical malpractice action is a claim against a licensed health-care provider based on the provider's alleged neglect or a breach of the standard of care in rendering mental health, medical, or nursing care.

A licensed health-care provider is defined as a person, corporation, or institution licensed by the state to provide mental health care, medical services, nursing services, or other health-related services. In mental health, the professionals include psychiatrists, psychologists, social workers, nurse practitioners, licensed professional counselors, and any other professional licensed by the state to provide mental health care. Medical and nursing providers include, but are not limited to, physicians, registered nurses, nurse practitioners, and licensed practical nurses.

Legal elements of a medical negligence claim

These elements, though differing slightly from state to state, depending on their statutory or common law basis required to support a medical negligence claim, are: 1) duty of care owed to the inmate; 2) breach of such duty; 3) proximate relationship between the breach of duty and the injury or death; and 4) damages.

The issue is whether a health-care provider deviated from the standard of care and such deviation had any direct connection (nexus) to the injury or death of the inmate. The deviation can be an act of commission, such as a wrong prescription, a premature removal from suicide watch, an abrupt discontinuation of medications, or similar acts that substantially impact the inmate's health. Acts of omission may include failure to evaluate obvious and substantial risk factors, failure to get information about past suicide attempts, failure to perform a suicide risk assessment, or similar omissions that place an inmate at risk.

To prevail in a malpractice claim, a plaintiff must prove that the health-care provider, by acts of commission or omission, failed to provide prudent care, given all the circumstances. Deviation from the standard of care can be assessed as ordinary negligence, gross negligence, not meeting the average practitioner standard or prudent practitioner standard. Ordinary negligence may include ordinary carelessness, laxity in care, or indifference, while gross negligence involves gross or egregious misconduct by the provider during care.

The average practitioner standard comprises applying a reasonable degree of knowledge and care an average provider exercises in diagnosing and treating an inmate. The prudent practitioner standard is what a prudent practitioner would do—utilizing his/her skill and knowledge in each situation under similar circumstances. A plaintiff must establish that the health-care provider failed to exercise that degree of care, skill, and learning expected of a prudent health-care provider of the specialization under the same or similar circumstances.

Thus, the prudent practitioner standard determines any deviation from the standard of care owed to the inmate. While simple negligence standards and gross negligence standards form the basis of a claim, most jurisdictions rely on the prudent practitioner standard to define the duty owed by the medical professional to the inmate patient.

There can be an error of fact or error of judgment. Should a provider fail to request records of an at-risk inmate from community sources or to have required lab tests performed, this is an error of fact. Should a provider gather relevant data, then make a misdiagnosis, this should be considered an error of judgment. In many states, error of judgment, such as negligent failure to diagnose, can be the basis of a medical malpractice claim. (See *Paynter v. Pro Assurance Wisconsin Ins. Co.*)[1]

Wrongful death action

A claim of wrongful death ordinarily relies on the same liability standards as a malpractice claim, and it often proceeds as a medical malpractice action against a health-care provider. The elements of a wrongful death claim are the same as for malpractice: breach of the standard of care in which the breach proximately cause the individual's death. The primary difference is the identity of the plaintiffs: for a malpractice claim, the typical plaintiff is the injured patient. But in a wrongful death case, the plaintiffs are the deceased patient's heirs and survivors, as discussed below.

Claimants

The claimants entitled to seek damages in a wrongful death case based on a medical negligence claim include the surviving spouse, children, or parents of the decedent or, if none survive, the decedent's estate. Usually, the plaintiff is the surviving child, spouse, parents, or the deceased's estate.

Experts in malpractice claim

Some jurisdictions stipulate the plaintiff must present a claim in a preliminary expert affidavit submitted in full compliance with the state statute. The testifying expert for the plaintiff must be qualified by experience, knowledge, education, and expertise to describe the standard of care and offer criticism against a defendant health-care provider.

The adversarial judicial process guarantees the defendant, (i.e., the health care provider or the organization), the right to establish, through the defendant's own expert witness' testimony, that the care and treatment provided to the decedent complied with the applicable standards of care and did not cause or contribute to the plaintiff's death or alleged injuries and damages.

Proximate cause

There are varying definitions of what constitutes proximate cause. Terms such as primary cause, substantial cause, "but for" and "case in fact" are interchangeably used in negligence lawsuits. Essentially, proximate cause is a legal cause of the injury or death: an act or event which the law recognizes as the primary cause of the negative outcome. It may not be the first act that set in motion the events that led to the injury—or the last act.

However, it is an act that caused foreseeable consequences in the absence of an intervening event. Foreseeability refers to whether a reasonable person would anticipate that his or her act or omission would cause an outcome, injury, or event in the natural course, unaltered by an intervening event. For instance, failure to place an actively suicidal inmate—with intent and plan—on suicide watch will constitute a legal cause for a negative result if the inmate commits suicide. Thus, failure to act can be a substantial factor in causing the injury or death. The substantial factor would then become the proximate cause. A plaintiff must show that the injury was the direct and natural consequence of the proximate cause.

Some jurisdictions use the "but-for" test. Such a test implies that had it not been for the omission or commission of the required level of care, a negative outcome would not have happened. If the negative outcome would not have occurred but for the negligent act by the defendant, proximate cause would be established.

NEGLIGENCE CLAIM AGAINST CORRECTIONAL OFFICERS
Correctional officers owe inmates a general duty to keep them safe from self-harm or harm by others when the officers have reason to appreciate such a risk. They should recognize inmate medical distress and act appropriately. Officers accomplish this by monitoring all inmates, but more specifically, by conducting inmate safety checks consistent with the facility's policy—that is, at 30 minutes or fewer intervals, preferably on an irregular basis.

They have a special duty in situations where an inmate is psychotic or under the influence of intoxication, causing him/her to be mentally unstable and unable to decide for his/her well-being. This special duty extends to inmates at risk for self-harm. A plaintiff may prevail if it can be established that an officer failed to recognize an inmate's potential risk and take appropriate action, where a reasonable officer would have both recognized the risk and acted. Such a failure can be a proximate cause of an inmate's suicide.

The key legal elements of a negligence claim are the same as in a malpractice claim: duty owed to the inmate, breach of duty, breach of duty as the proximate cause of injury or death. A negligence claim does not require an officer to have actual knowledge of an inmate's particular suicide vulnerability, but the mere knowledge that if he/she does not take a specific action that includes standard procedures and practice, harm will probably result to the inmate. The standard of proof required to prevail in a negligence case is the preponderance of the evidence (more likely than not). This is a much lower standard of proof than a deliberate indifference claim.

In *Hott v. Hennepin County*[2] the Eighth Circuit determined that an officer owed a general duty to protect an inmate from self-harm by performing safety checks every half an hour consistent with the county jail policy. Failing to do so, the officer should face a negligence lawsuit.

Philip Hott, an eighteen-year-old man, hanged himself in his cell at Adult Detention Center (ADC) in Hennepin County, Minnesota, during early morning hours on January 21, 1996, using a torn bedsheet. Deputy Rieder was on duty for the unique needs section of the ADC that night. His log indicated that he conducted an inmate safety check consistent with the Center's policy approximately every 30 minutes. He last logged in at 5:48 a.m. and stated, "all appears ok."

The medical examiner opined that Hott was likely dead for hours before his body was discovered. He was seated at the foot of his bed during the period when Rieder repeatedly performed the checks and documented in the log that all appeared normal. Several inmates at the Center reported that the checks were not regularly conducted.

Mr. Hott's estate sued Deputy Reider and his supervisor, asserting claims of negligence by failing to protect the safety of the inmate under Minnesota state law. The issue was whether Rieder had breached a general duty to conduct inmate safety checks to reduce the risk of suicide.

Under Minnesota law, "the plaintiff's evidentiary burden on the issue of proximate cause in an action for negligence is to show that it is more likely than not that an act or omission was a substantial factor in bringing about the result." In reversing the summary judgment on the issue of negligence, the Eighth Circuit opined that the plaintiff was "entitled to proceed at trial if evidence is sufficient to support a jury finding that Rieder's breach of that duty was a proximate cause of Hott's death." The case was remanded to the district court for further proceedings concerning the negligence claim against Rieder.

The court recognized two incidental findings relevant to suicide prevention in jails: 1) staggered-time checks are an effective means of both detecting and deterring inmate suicide attempts; and 2) training officers on suicide prevention policy has been an effective tool to prevent suicides. The court noted, "The record does not, however, contain any evidence to suggest that any negligence on Rieder's part was due to Hennepin County's failure to train or supervise him. If anything, the low incidence of inmate suicide at the ADC suggests quite the opposite conclusion, for it implies that ADC's policies and procedures are, on the whole, quite successful in preventing inmate suicide."

CONTRIBUTORY NEGLIGENCE AND ASSUMPTION OF RISK
Contributory negligence is defined as the plaintiff's failure to take reasonable care for his care and safety. Assumption of risk is a defense based on the notion that the plaintiff consented to the defendant's conduct, which annuls the theory of negligence.[3] The party asserting contributory negligence has the burden of proof of such a defense. The standard of proof is the preponderance of the evidence. The legal elements include only duty, breach of duty, and causation. Contributory negligence bars plaintiffs from recovery if they are found to be negligent.

Courts have begun to use the principle of comparative fault which, arguably, requires the court to factor the decedent's conduct in the apportionment of liability. The Tennessee

Supreme Court, in *McIntyre v. Balentine*,[4] opined in 1992 that "it is time to abandon the outmoded and unjust common law doctrine of contributory negligence and adopt in its place a system of comparative fault." Today, some jurisdictions use comparative fault principle. However, many jurisdictions continue to recognize the contributory negligence of the deceased.

There are two types of comparative fault: pure and modified. In pure comparative fault jurisdictions, the plaintiff can still recover damages from the defendant, minus his or her percentage of responsibility. For example, if the plaintiff is 70% at fault, he/she can recover 30% of his/her damages. In modified comparative fault states, the plaintiff should be either 50% or less at fault. It depends on the jurisdiction. Some say the plaintiff must be less than 50% at fault to recover, whereas some allow recovery where the plaintiff and defendant are equally at fault.

In some jurisdictions, contributory negligence cannot be a defense in medical negligence or suicide in custody. Courts have long recognized that there can be no contributory negligence where "the defendant's duty of care includes preventing the self-abusive or self-destructive acts that caused the plaintiff's injuries."[5] In *Cowan v. Doering*, the Supreme Court of New Jersey held that "[T]he acts which plaintiff's mental illness allegedly caused him to commit were the very acts which defendants had a duty to prevent, and these same acts, cannot as a matter of law, constitute contributory negligence."[6]

In *Gregoire v. City of Oak Harbor*,[7] the Supreme Court of Washington State held that contributory negligence defense cannot be used in a custodial suicidal death.[7] In this case, the court recognized that "jailers have a special relationship with inmates, creating an affirmative duty to provide for inmate health, welfare, and safety." The court further found that because the jailers have this special relationship, a claim of contributory negligence was inappropriate in a case of suicide in jail.

Edward Gregoire showed a range of inappropriate behaviors, including violence and crying, and made irrational statements, that is, asking the officers to shoot him at the time of arrest and booking. Shortly after he was booked in at Oak Harbor jail, he hanged himself. He was left alone in a cell. The jail officials performed no suicide screening. Tanya Gregoire, the personal representative of his estate, sued the jail for negligence in his death.

During the trial, the trial court read jury instructions on the assumption of risk and contributory negligence. The jury found that the jail was negligent, but it was not the proximate cause of death; rather that Gregoire took his own life. The appeals court affirmed the lower court decision. The Washington State Supreme Court reversed the decision, ruling that contributory negligence is inappropriate in inmate suicide. The court opined that the affirmative duty to protect the inmate cannot be nullified by the inmate's assumption of the risk of death by suicide.

There are certain murky situations in jails and prisons where contributory negligence may be considered. For instance, if an inmate consumes illicit drugs and commits suicide by hanging in an altered mental state, can the defendant utilize contributory negligence defense? To the extent that an inmate illicitly consumes any mind-altering medication or substance that impaired his judgment, he assumes the risk. He is likely at fault for consuming illegal drugs which caused or contributed to his death. It is common for inmates with antisocial personality disorder and impulsivity to attempt suicide and suffer death or injuries. Would the defendant prevail by using contributory negligence defense in the event a survivor sues the jail? Other situations may include refusal of treatment and medications or withholding pertinent information.

DELIBERATE INDIFFERENCE

History and concept

In 1976, the U.S. Supreme Court held that prisoners have a right to treatment for serious medical needs.

The term "deliberate indifference" originated in *Estelle v. Gamble.*[8] An inmate in the Texas prison system complained of inadequate medical care for back pain (a bale of cotton fell on him). Although a doctor examined him and prescribed pain medication, the inmate claimed that he was not given appropriate medication, and, therefore, he received inadequate medical care, violating his Eighth Amendment rights. He was also known to be someone who fabricated medical complaints. In this case, the U.S. Supreme Court opined that he was not given "inadequate medical treatment" and that the Texas system did not violate his Eighth Amendment rights. Although the Court did not offer a precise definition of what constituted deliberate indifference, the court opined that "[d]eliberate indifference to the prisoners' serious medical need constituted unnecessary and wanton infliction of pain." More significantly, however, Justice Thurgood Marshall opined that mere negligence or medical malpractice does not amount to deliberate indifference. To violate Eighth Amendment rights, the indifference must offend evolving standards of decency. The prisoner must allege "acts of omission, sufficiently harmful, to evidence deliberate indifference to serious medical needs."

Serious medical need

A critical concept in understanding deliberate indifference is "serious medical need." In *Bowring v. Godwin* (1977)[9] the Fourth Circuit Court of Appeals emphasized the lack of underlying distinction between the right to medical care for physical illness and its psychological or psychiatric counterpart. In Bowring, the court further noted that the medical necessity determines the seriousness test. If treatment is not provided after a mental illness is diagnosed, and such a lack of treatment will result in unnecessary and wanton infliction of pain, this constitutes a serious medical need.

Over the last four decades, the courts have attempted to define "serious medical need." In 2006, in *Gobert v. Caldwell*[10] the court indicated that "A serious medical need is one for which treatment has been recommended or for which the need is so apparent that even laypeople would recognize that care is required." The courts did not specify the kind or level of treatment, but it is understood that the treatment should be adequate but not necessarily what is most desirable or the best care.

Farmer v. Brennan (1994)

The legal concept of deliberate indifference was clarified in a landmark Supreme Court case, *Farmer v. Brennan.*[11] Farmer, a transsexual inmate, alleged that he was beaten and raped by another inmate in his cell and the prison officials were deliberately indifferent because they failed to ensure his personal security. The court found that an official is deliberately indifferent if he "knew of and disregarded an excessive risk to inmate health or safety. The official must both be aware of facts from which the inference could be drawn that a substantial risk of serious harm exists, and he must also draw the inference."

In this case, writing for the majority, Justice David Souter defined deliberate indifference as "reckless disregard," indicating an intent to deprive the prisoner of his or her security, a standard higher than mere negligence. Justice Souter further stated that deliberate indifference is a mental state more blameworthy than negligence. He positioned it somewhere between negligence at one end and purpose or intent at the other, amounting to "recklessness." The plaintiff is required to show that the defendants (prison officials or health-care professionals) "knew" (had actual knowledge as opposed to should have known) of the serious medical need and nonetheless disregarded the "excessive risk to inmate's health or safety."

An example would be when a psychiatrist in private practice in the outside community, after diagnosing a patient with depression and assessing suicide risk, prescribes a 30-day supply of tricyclic antidepressant at a daily dose of 100 mg. The patient takes the entire supply and kills himself. Here, a claim of negligence can be made because the prescriber should have known that a supply of over 3000 mg of tricyclics would be lethal. Though the prescription would be appropriate to treat the patient's depression, a prescription that supplies a suicidal patient with a lethal amount breaches the standard of care.

In prison, the same situation may not be considered deliberately indifferent if the psychiatrist prescribes the 100 mg daily dose in a facility where medication is administered daily. The prisoner would not have a large supply unless he/she cheeks his/her medication and hoards it until they've accumulated a lethal amount. In this situation, the psychiatrist defendant would legitimately claim that a reasonably appropriate dose of tricyclics was prescribed to relieve the prisoner's suffering and pain.

If a psychiatrist knew about a prisoner's recent near-lethal suicide attempt, yet prescribes an antidepressant with lethal impact—such as a tricyclic as noted above—this may amount to deliberate indifference: The psychiatrist knew about the suicidal risk and failed to act appropriately.

Post-Farmer Period

Although the Eighth Amendment applies only to convicted persons, pretrial detainees are entitled to the same basic protections under the Fourteenth Amendment's due process clause.[12] About half the federal appellate courts apply the same legal standards to deliberate indifference claims brought under either the Eighth or Fourteenth Amendments. However, all the other courts of appeal applied a lower standard of reasonable care to pretrial detainees, consistent with provisions of the Fourth Amendment.

If a detainee is first brought to jail, and a court hasn't yet ruled that there is probable cause to hold him/her, then their right to medical care stems from the Fourth Amendment, which prohibits unreasonable seizures. The applicable standard here is whether the care provided to the detainee was reasonable, meaning the plaintiff need not show that the care provider knew of the problem and ignored it; it would be sufficient to show that the provider should have known, and the care provided was not reasonable.

Some federal circuit courts of appeal have held that a pretrial detainee's right to medical care is analogous to the Eighth Amendment, others, to the Fourth Amendment. The U.S. Supreme Court has not yet weighed in on this "split" among the circuits.

Various courts have defined deliberate indifference. Perhaps, the court in *Crayton v. Quarterman*[13] provided the most succinct and workable definition of deliberate indifference. The court stated: "You knew there was a substantial risk of serious harm to the inmate, you knew it right then, and you did nothing about it." Failure to act where prison officials know a substantial risk of serious harm to inmate health or safety constitutes deliberate indifference.

A prison physician examined an inmate who had recently attempted suicide. After assessing the current risk, he found that the prisoner was at risk but did nothing further—he did not place the prisoner on suicide watch, move him to an acute stabilization unit, or commit him involuntarily to a mental health unit even though the inmate refused medical care. The inmate took his life a short time later. In this scenario, the physician knew the inmate was likely to harm himself; yet he did nothing about it.

To prevail on an Eighth Amendment claim "a prisoner is not required to show that his complaints were 'literally ignored' but only that the defendants' responses were so plainly inappropriate as to permit the inference that the defendants intentionally or recklessly disregarded his needs."[14]

In *Elliot v. Jones*[15] the court emphasized first the importance of awareness of facts from which an inference of risk can be drawn, and second "actually" drawing the inference that substantial harm exists. In other words, first, there must be facts showing an inmate's likelihood of committing suicide. Second, the prison officials must know the facts. Finally, the official must draw an inference based on his awareness of facts. In *Thompson v. Upshur*[16] the court went a step further by emphasizing that the official's response must show that the official subjectively intended that harm will occur. However, in *Cavalieri v. Shepard*[12] the court noted that the "plaintiff need not show that a prison official acted or failed to act believing that harm actually would befall an inmate; it is enough that the official acted or failed to act despite his knowledge of a substantial risk of serious harm."

In *Petties v. Carter*[17] the Seventh Circuit stated that once a prison official or health-care provider is aware of a substantial risk of serious harm, including self-harm, the next step is to assess the official's/provider's response. The court further noted: "To determine if a prison official acted with deliberate indifference, we look into his or her subjective state of mind. For a prison official's acts or omissions to constitute deliberate indifference, a plaintiff does not need to show that the official intended harm or believed that harm would occur, but showing mere negligence is not enough. Medical malpractice does not become a constitutional violation merely because the victim is a prisoner . . . Even objective recklessness—failing to act in the face of an unjustifiably high risk that is so obvious that it should be known—is insufficient to make out a claim. Instead, the Supreme Court has instructed us that a plaintiff must provide evidence that an official actually knew of and disregarded a substantial risk of harm. Officials can avoid liability by proving they were unaware even of an obvious risk to inmate health or safety."

Regarding pretrial detainees, the Ninth Circuit held that "claims for violations of the right to adequate medical care 'brought by pretrial detainees against individual defendants under the Fourteenth Amendment' must be evaluated under an objective deliberate indifference standard" as opposed to subjective indifference standard.[18] Prior to decision in *Castro v. Cnty. of L.A.* [19] the Ninth Circuit noted that: "All conditions of confinement claims, including claims for inadequate medical care, were analyzed under a subjective deliberate indifference standard whether brought by a convicted prisoner under the Eighth Amendment or pretrial detainee under the Fourteenth Amendment."

The court noted in *Gordon v. Cnty of Orange*[18] that a pretrial detainee's medical claim against an individual defendant under due process clause of the Fourteenth Amendment, emphasizing the objective indifference standard includes: (1) the defendant made an intentional decision under which the plaintiff was held; (2) those conditions put the plaintiff at substantial risk of suffering serious harm; (3) the defendant did not take reasonable available measures to abate that risk, even though a reasonable official in the circumstances would have appreciated the high degree of risk involved—making the conduct of the defendant's conduct obvious; and (4) by not taking such measures, the defendant caused the plaintiff's injuries.

The Seventh Circuit most recently held in *Pittman by & through Hamilton v. County of Madison, Illinois*[20] that the jury must answer two questions. First, it must decide whether the "defendants acted purposefully, knowingly, or perhaps even recklessly." Second, it must determine whether the defendants' actions were "objectively reasonable . . . If the defendants "were aware" that their actions would be harmful, then they acted "purposefully" or "knowingly"; if they were not necessarily "aware" but nevertheless "strongly suspected" that their actions would lead to harmful results, then they acted "recklessly."

NEGLIGENCE VS DELIBERATE INDIFFERENCE

Justice Thurgood Marshall (1976) eloquently pointed out that deliberate indifference is more than mere negligence or medical negligence. Justice David Souter (1994) defined deliberate indifference as a state of mind more blameworthy than negligence.

Earlier in 1986, the U.S. Supreme Court in *Daniels v. Williams*[21] held negligent conduct per se does not rise to the level of a constitutional violation. Later, the Fifth Circuit ruled that deliberate indifference cannot be inferred from a negligent or grossly negligent response to a substantial risk of harm—*Hare v. City of Corinth*[22] and *Thompson v. Upshur.*[16]

Some argue what is required is good faith practice or reasonable efforts to avert the anticipated harm.[22] However, significant distinction exists between a negligent, or grossly negligent act, and a constitutional violation, as noted in the historical court decisions.

PROFESSIONAL JUDGMENT STANDARD

If a medical decision involving diagnosis, monitoring and treatment of an inmate at risk forms the basis of a deliberate indifference claim, the standard of professional judgment is often used. A *substantial departure* [emphasis added] from the accepted professional judgment, practice, and standard is required to support a claim. What is substantial departure is yet to be defined; however, medical professionals should know. A medical provider is expected to exercise reasonable and appropriate professional judgment in matters involving suicide risk mitigation.

In 1996, in *Estate of Cole v. Fromm*[23] the Seventh Circuit has explained the professional judgment standard this way: "The question then becomes how 'obvious' a risk must be, or how 'erroneous' a medical professional's treatment decision must be, such that a jury may infer subjective awareness of the risk in a medical treatment case. The answer is that deliberate indifference may be inferred based upon a medical professional's erroneous treatment decision only when the medical professional's decision is such a substantial departure from accepted professional judgment, practice, or standards as to demonstrate that the person responsible did not base the decision on such a judgment."

In a 2016 case, *Petties v. Carter*,[17] the Seventh Circuit emphasized professional judgment in treatment decision if it is a substantial departure from accepted practice: "[A] medical professional's treatment decision must be such a substantial departure from accepted professional judgment, practice, or standards as to demonstrate that the person responsible did not base the decision on such a judgment."

SUICIDE VULNERABILITY

For the expert, the concept of an inmate's particular suicide vulnerability may provide a reasonable basis in providing opinions to the court.

An inmate's [substantial probability] [likelihood] of engaging in serious self-harm or suicide would constitute a serious medical need, requiring active intervention. The court in *Palakovic v. Wetzel*[24] established that: 1) the individual should have a particular vulnerability to suicide, meaning that there was a "strong likelihood," rather than a mere possibility, that suicide would be attempted; 2) the prison official knew or should have known of the individual's particular vulnerability; and 3) the official acted with reckless or deliberate indifference, meaning something beyond mere negligence, to the individual's particular vulnerability. As opposed to the Farmer case, the court expanded the required element to include the "prison officials should have known" the vulnerability.

In *Estate of Kempf v. Washington City*[25] the court determined that "the (decedent) posed a significant suicide risk at the time he was booked and remained so throughout the confinement at (prison); and the placement of the (decedent) in a cell with known anchor points with bedsheets and clothing, knowing his obvious and substantial risk, amounted to deliberate indifference."

The presence of obvious and substantial risk factors often determines an inmate's suicide vulnerability. Typically, the risk factors include active suicidal ideation with intent and plan; presence of diagnosed mental disorder, particularly depression; anxiety, and agitation with hopelessness; a history of nearly lethal suicide attempt within the preceding six months to a year of the final act; and alcohol or opiate intoxication and withdrawal. In denying a summary judgment motion by the defendant in *Lewis v. Northumberland County*[26] the court emphasized Lewis' most recent serious suicide attempt, opiate withdrawal, premature discontinuation of suicide watches, mental status changes, and his classification as high risk for suicide as obvious and substantial risk factors.

It may appear that the standard in the corrections environment is strict liability: (i.e., if an inmate dies in custody, the facility security and medical staff are liable because they had a duty to prevent custodial suicides). However, whether prison officials and providers assume the inmate's duty to avoid self-harm is more nuanced.

Charles Williams, in a law review article,[27] stated that "[t]wo key facts are common in the cases finding that third parties have assumed a suicidal person's duty of care: 1) the defendant exercised custody or control over the suicide victim; and 2) the defendant knew or had reason to know that the suicide victim was a danger to himself. So the duty to prevent the self-harm of a person in custody never arises if prison officials had no reason to believe the inmate posed a specific, rather than generalized, suicide risk."

Of course, they could still be responsible for the custodial suicide if they failed to do things, like performing an intake suicide assessment, that would have alerted them to the risk that the deceased inmate was at heightened risk of suicide.

TYPICAL ALLEGATION IN A DELIBERATE INDIFFERENCE LAWSUIT

The typical allegation in a deliberate indifference complaint focuses on how the facility officials and health-care providers intentionally disregarded an inmate's serious medical need. The deliberate indifference standard requires that an individual defendant's actions or failure to act must be proved for the claim to prevail. While "a total deprivation of care is not a necessary condition for finding a constitutional violation, grossly incompetent or inadequate care can also constitute deliberate indifference."[28]

MONELL CLAIMS

Another type of §1983 allegation targets the governmental entity that operates the facility or a private company that operates the facility or provides health care under government contract. These lawsuits focus on the conduct and decisions of the institutional policymakers and often involve claims of poor staffing and lack of staff training as factors causing and contributing to inmate suicide. Such claims have their origin in *Monell v. Department of Social Services, of the City of New York.*[29] Monell claims may include the following:

1. Widespread denial of adequate and proper access to mental health services
2. Inadequate psychiatric treatment
3. Lack of compliance with suicide prevention measures
4. A pattern of inadequate suicide watch and monitoring
5. Inadequate crisis monitoring
6. Understaffing resulting in deprivation of adequate mental health and medical care
7. Lack of staff training
8. Inadequate supervisions

It is often said that some practices by correctional or mental health officials at a facility would become so well settled that they become de facto policy (custom) at the facility, giving the appearance that it has been approved by the policymaker.

For instance, routinely placing mentally ill inmates in solitary confinement—even if a policy prohibits it—becomes the custom at that facility, placing inmates at risk of harm. Another example would be housing an inmate in the second tier of the jail despite that inmate's history of jumping and a policy restricting such housing; or repeatedly failing to place an inmate on suicide watch despite knowing that the inmate had been suicidal during several episodes of incarceration.

There are several key elements pertinent to Monell claims:

1. *There must be a de facto organizational custom, policy, or practice.*
2. *The organization's policymaker must know of the deficient custom, policy, or practice and fail to correct it.* The sheriff of a jail or the chief administrator of a prison or relevant policymaker must know that deficient procedures exist and fail to correct them. *Dixon v. County of Cook*[30] established that a plaintiff could prevail on a Monell claim only if "a policy-making official knows about [the deficiencies in procedure] and fails to correct them." In *Gable v. City of Chicago*[31] the court noted the plaintiff must show that the policymakers were "deliberately indifferent as to [the] known or obvious consequences" of the policy. In other words, they must have been aware of the risk created by the custom or practice and must have failed to take appropriate steps to protect the decedent (plaintiff).

3. *Absence of policy.* In situations where rules or regulations are required to remedy a potentially dangerous practice, the facility's failure to make such a policy may also be actionable.[32, 33]

4. *Pervasiveness of unlawful practice.* In the absence of a defective, officially adopted policy, custom, or practice, widespread existence of a custom may be shown by the frequency and pervasive occurrence of an unlawful practice. To prove the existence of a widespread custom, a "plaintiff must introduce evidence demonstrating that the unlawful practice was so pervasive that acquiescence on the part of policymakers was apparent and amounted to a policy decision. This requires more than a showing of one or two missteps."[30]

The Seventh Circuit has remarked that "there is no clear consensus as to how frequently . . . conduct must occur to impose Monell liability."[34] However, it falls to a plaintiff to demonstrate that there is a de facto policy at issue rather than simply a random event. "[T]this may take the form of an implicit policy or a gap in expressed policies" or "a series of violations to lay the premise of deliberate indifference." In the *Woodward v. Correctional Medical Services*[35] decision, the court noted that the provider does not get a "one free suicide" pass. Here, there was a direct link between Correctional Medical Services'(CMS) policies and Justin Farver's suicide (1998). That no one in the past committed suicide simply shows that CMS was fortunate, not that it wasn't deliberately indifferent.

It is the province of the jury to decide whether the evidence supports that the facility had a widespread practice that resulted in the alleged constitutional harm.

Monell Claim on Training and Supervision

Training and supervision of the staff are interrelated. Failure to train and inadequate supervision are often claimed to support a Monell claim. In *City of Canton v. Harris*[36] the U.S. Supreme Court held that "the inadequacy of police training may serve as the basis for §1983 liability only where the failure to train amounts to deliberate indifference to the rights of persons with whom the police come into contact." The Court of Appeals for the Seventh Circuit has recognized a deliberate indifference claim premised on a lack of supervision, saying, "This proof can take the form of either 1) failure to provide adequate training in light of foreseeable consequences, or 2) failure to act in response to repeated complaints of constitutional violations by its officers."[37] Lack of oversight on the part of policymakers may also demonstrate deliberate indifference.

In *Flores v. City of S. Bend,*[38] a recent Fourth Amendment case, the Seventh Circuit opined that the City of South Bend can be found liable for failure to train its police officers to refrain from reckless driving that caused the death of Ms. Sorida Flores, who was tragically killed in a police chase. Although this is not a deliberate indifference case involving serious medical need, the principle of failure to train its employees can support §1983 liability.

To prevail in a Monell claim related to training, the plaintiff must show the government or health-care entity's training of their professionals was grossly inadequate; they knew about it; and they took no remedial action to prevent serious harm to the inmates.

QUALIFIED IMMUNITY

Qualified immunity is intended to balance two important values: "the public interest in deterring unlawful conduct and providing compensation for victims who suffer constitutional violations versus the cost of subjecting public officials to a lawsuit"—both the actual cost and the social cost of litigation.[39]

A correctional official employed by a governmental entity may assert an entitlement to qualified immunity. When applicable, a qualified immunity defense entitles an officer "not to stand trial or face the other burdens of litigation."[40, 41]

To stave off a qualified immunity defense, the plaintiff must establish that a constitutional violation occurred and that the conduct in question was clearly established as a constitutional violation at the time it was committed. The Supreme Court noted that a constitutional right is "clearly established" when it would be clear to a reasonable public official that his or her conduct was unlawful in the context of the situation confronted.[40]

An official is entitled to immunity from civil suit if the facts of the case reveal no constitutional violation by the official.[40, 42]

Cavalieri v. Shepard[12] is one of many suicide-in-jail cases in which the Seventh Circuit has addressed the issue of qualified immunity. On June 4, 1998, Stephen Cavalieri kidnapped his former girlfriend and held her hostage. During the standoff, which lasted for several hours, Cavalieri's mother informed the officers that her son was suicidal and needed to be hospitalized. After he was taken into custody, his girlfriend informed the officers that he'd threatened to kill himself during the hostage situation.

After Cavalieri arrived at the city jail, he met with Officer Donald Shepard for approximately one hour. During the meeting, the officer granted Cavalieri's request to speak with a mental health counselor. However, no meeting with a mental health professional took place because Cavalieri was transferred from the city jail to the county jail. After the transfer, Officer Shepard remained involved in the case. He met with Cavalieri's mother, who again shared her concerns about her son's suicide potential. The officer, after speaking with Cavalieri on the phone, determined that he was not suicidal. Cavalieri was placed in a holding cell in the county jail to await further booking. Cavalieri was never placed on suicide watch, either in the city jail or county jail. He never informed the officers at the county jail that he was suicidal. He attempted to strangle himself with a telephone cord in the county jail, which left him in a permanent vegetative state.

The district court denied the defendant's motion for summary judgment in which the defendant claimed an entitlement to qualified immunity. The defendant filed an appeal. The Seventh Circuit affirmed the trial court decision and stated that there is "no doubt that [the right to be free from deliberate indifference to suicide] was clearly established prior to his 1998 suicide attempt"—implying that the defendant probably violated the decedent's constitutional rights, knowing his suicide risk.

CONTRACT EMPLOYEE VS STATE/COUNTY EMPLOYEE
A crucial element in a §1983 case is that the defendant was working "under color of state law" at the time of the constitutional

violation. Correctional officials employed by state departments of corrections or county jails are liable if there is evidence of constitutional violation, as noted previously, although they are obviously working under color of state law.

However, many privately employed physicians and psychiatrists work as contractors to provide medical and psychiatric services. The question of whether these private providers can be found liable under §1983 was addressed by the U.S. Supreme Court, which ruled that delivery of medical treatment to prisoner by a contracted health-care provider qualifies as state action for purposes of 42 U.S.C. §1983.[43] In *West v. Atkins*, the Supreme Court held that "[T]he State [has] a constitutional duty to provide adequate medical treatment to those in its custody," and constitutional claims may be brought against medical care providers, regardless of "the precise terms of [their] employment," when they "voluntarily assume that obligation by contract."

In *West*, a prisoner claimed that an orthopedic physician employed part-time on contract gave him inadequate medical services at a prison in North Carolina. The district court entered a judgment that the contract physician was not acting "under the color of the law" because he was not an employee of the state. The court of appeals affirmed the decision. However, the U.S. Supreme Court reversed the decision by declaring, "A physician who is under contract with the state to provide medical services to inmates at a state prison hospital on a part-time basis act 'under the color of the law' within the meaning of U.S. 1983, when he treats an inmate."

ADA-BASED CLAIMS

Title II of the Americans with Disabilities Act, 42 U.S.C. §12132 et seq., (hereinafter "ADA") provides "no qualified individual with a disability shall, by reason of such disability, be excluded from participation in or be denied the benefits of the services, programs, or activities of a public entity, or be subjected to discrimination by such entity." It bars public entities, including prisons, from "excluding the disabled from participating in or benefiting from a public program, activity, or service 'solely by reason of disability.' " An ADA claim centers on whether the disabled individual allegedly was treated differently or whether "other non-disabled individuals without the disability were treated more favorably."[44]

A mentally ill, suicidal inmate could be considered disabled under ADA. A correctional facility's failure to provide reasonable accommodations such as increased safety checks or housing in a medical unit for close observation or failure to train the staff on protective aspects of ADA may form the basis of an ADA-based lawsuit. Such a claim is often made on the premise that the employer or the government entity responsible for a facility owes a duty to ensure the health and safety of the potentially at-risk inmates and that such safety would not be compromised by the actions or inactions of the facility's employees.

An ADA-based claim must allege that the plaintiff was excluded from or discriminated against regarding services, programs, or activities because of disability.[45]

A search on www.casetext.com database using the following string of words: Suicide /p ADA /p AND/ deliberate/ Indifference/ (jails and prisons) yielded eighty-three case decisions involving ADA claims as an issue. All ADA claims were made in conjunction with deliberate indifference claims. With "deliberate indifference" excluded, I found an additional one hundred cases. I have selected a few cases to highlight issues related to ADA-based claims. They include:

1. inadequate medical care;
2. denial of treatment;
3. discriminatory practices involving screening and monitoring;
4. failure to train the staff; and
5. cell assignment.

Various court decisions show that the failure to provide or attend to inmate medical needs or inadequate medical care does not support a violation of the ADA.[46, 47, 48] In the case of *Bearden v. McKeithen*[46] on March 22, 2009, Maureen Bearden committed suicide by hanging in the Bay County Jail. She was booked into the jail in January 2009. She had a history of numerous suicide attempts and placement on suicide watch several times between 2006 and 2008 during her prior incarcerations in the same jail.

In this case, the court considered whether Bearden was "denied the benefits of the services, programs, or activities" of the Bay County Jail. The plaintiff (James Bearden), as personal representative of Ms. Bearden, alleged that Ms. Bearden, "because of her lack of treatment and adequate supervision, was denied certain opportunities that other inmates enjoyed, such as the opportunity to interact with other inmates, form friendships, move at liberty within set bounds, make phone calls, use educational facilities, and engage in religious activities."

The court in *Bearden v. McKeithen* noted that "a prison would not violate the ADA simply failing to attend to the medical needs of its disabled prisoners," relying on *Bryant v. Madigan*.[48] The court ruled that the failure to provide adequate medical care for Ms. Bearden's mental illness is not by itself an ADA violation.

During detention at the Callaway County Jail, Cassandra Cox made a statement on February 26, 2016, that she wanted to die.[49] She refused lunch and dinner and a shower. She was then placed in a cell on observational status and provided with a green suicide prevention suit. While under observation, Cox was scheduled to be observed in regular intervals from February 26, 2016, until her departure from the jail on February 28, 2016.

On February 27, her father requested that she be transferred to a psychiatric unit, but the officer in charge did not think it was needed because she did not appear "to be crazy." On February 28, 2016, she became unconscious and did not respond to ammonia inhalants. CPR was started, and she was transferred to a hospital.

Cox sued, alleging that deliberate indifference to her medical need caused her to have a heart attack and brain damage. She also alleged state law negligence, Monell liability, and violation of ADA. Cox claimed that Callaway County discriminated against her by (1) failing to accommodate her disability by not screening for mental illness or educating officers regarding mental illness; (2) failing to adopt a policy to protect people with mental illness; (3) discriminating against her in a mental health crisis situation by not accommodating her disability; (4) failing to modify its programs to accommodate the needs of persons with mental impairments; and (5) failing to train and supervise deputies regarding individuals with mental impairments.

Courts have opined that deliberate indifference was the appropriate standard for showing intentional discrimination in this type of cases.[50] Evidence of intentional discrimination of an inmate because of disability is required for compensatory damages."[51] Under the deliberate indifference standard, intentional discrimination "does not require a showing of personal ill will or animosity toward the disabled person," but instead can be "inferred from a defendant's deliberate indifference to the strong likelihood that pursuit of its questioned policies will probably result in a violation of federal law."[51]

Cox argued that the deliberate indifference standard did not apply to her claims, but the court disagreed. The court found that "each of these alleged acts of discrimination is inherently claims of inadequate medical care which cannot be the basis of an ADA claim."

In *Smizer v. Standard*[52] the court reached the same conclusion. Wendell Smizer alleged that, from March 23, 2015, to April 6, 2016, during his detention at the Fulton County Jail, he repeatedly asked to speak with a mental health professional and requested mental health treatment. Officer Doug Lafary withheld treatment, allegedly demanding a confession for a crime that Smizer did not commit. Lafary also requested payment from Smizer or his family for consultation. Lafary placed Smizer in a suicide watch cell, which worsened his mental condition. Smizer attempted suicide twice and went on a hunger strike. Fulton County Sheriff Jeff Standard was reportedly aware of this situation and took no action.

The court found that, under the ADA, the claim was not viable because the ADA does not provide a remedy for the failure to treat a condition. The court relied on *Bryant v. Madigan*, which indicated a "prison simply failing to attend to the medical needs of its disabled prisoners does not violate the ADA."

Inadequate medical care cannot be the basis of an ADA claim. In *A.H. v. St. Louis County*[47] the plaintiff argued that the decedent could have enjoyed various benefits of jail life but for "lack of treatment and adequate supervision" and further claimed that he was not given proper medication and security monitoring that could have prevented him from committing suicide. The court found that the basic issue was one of treatment but not discrimination. Therefore, dismissal of ADA claim by the lower court was affirmed by the Eighth Circuit Court of Appeals.

In *Trevino v. Woodbury County Jail*,[53] a wheelchair-bound inmate claimed discrimination for his placement in an isolation cell. The court granted a summary judgment to the jail defendant, finding that the inmate was put in an isolated cell for "his safety because he would have been an easy target for violent inmates in the general population." Likewise, placement in a quiet room for close monitoring of a suicidal inmate cannot be found to be discriminatory.

In contrast, *Arenas v. Georgia Department of Corrections*[54] is a case in which the plaintiff's ADA-based claim for inmate suicide survived a motion for a summary judgment. The decedent, Richard Tavara, had severe mental illness and a history of prior suicide attempt, which the defendants knew. He was housed in a solitary cell that had access to a fire extinguisher sprinkler on the ceiling—a known anchor for hanging.

The court noted that Tavara's disability was not properly accommodated by placing him in an appropriate cell. The claim was materially different from inadequate treatment because he was not provided with a reasonable housing accommodation considering his disability. As such, to the extent that the plaintiff's claim is premised on the failure to provide certain accommodations related to Tavara's disability, such as an appropriate cell assignment, then this claim "survives."

CONCLUSION

The standard of proof for medical negligence or other types of negligence claims is preponderance of the evidence, but deliberate indifference is a higher legal standard.

As of now, court decisions established substantial clarity regarding the basis of deliberate indifference claims. Although courts consider whether the prison officials knew or should have known the "particular vulnerability to suicide," significant unresolved issues exist regarding the nature of objective facts, clinical or otherwise, from which an official can be said to have drawn an inference of such vulnerability.

The second component of a deliberate indifference claim is based on whether an official intentionally disregarded, by acts of commission or omission, or failed to respond reasonably to, the suicide vulnerability of an inmate that was obvious.

Although proof of this latter component is predicated upon the subjective mental state of an official, its existence can be objectively determined by evaluating the actions the official took or failed to take to deal with the inmate's risk.

ADA-based claims related to inmate suicide rarely survive because of the inherent difficulty to prove discrimination in treatment. The applicable standard the court has relied on is that of deliberate indifference.

REFERENCES

1. Paynter v. ProAssurance Wis. Ins. Co., 387 Wis. 2d 278 (Wis. 2019)
2. Hott ex rel. Estate of Hott v. Hennepin County, 260 F.3d 901 (8th Cir. 2001)
3. Hylton, K. *Contributory Negligence and Assumption of Risk.*" In *Tort Law: A Modern Perspective. Cambridge University Press* (2016) 147–169
4. McIntyre v. Balentine, 833 S.W.2d 52 (Tenn. 1992)
5. Mulhern v. Catholic Health Initiatives, 799 N.W.2d 104 (Iowa 2011)
6. Cowan v. Doering, 111 N.J. 451 (1988)
7. Gregoire v. City of Oak Harbor, 170 Wn. 2d 628 (Wash. 2010)
8. Estelle v. Gamble, 429 U.S. 97 (1976)
9. Bowring v. Godwin, 551 F.2d 44 (4th Cir. 1977)
10. Gobert v. Caldwell, 463 F.3d 339 (5th Cir. 2006)
11. Farmer v. Brennan, 511 U.S. 825 (1994)
12. Cavalieri v. Shepard, 321 F.3d 616 (7th Cir. 2003)
13. Crayton v. Quarterman, 2009 U.S. Dist. LEXIS 103709 (N.D. Tex. Oct. 14, 2009)

14. Hayes v. Snyder, 546 F.3d 516, 524 (7th Cir. 2008) (quoting Sherrod v. Lingle, 223 F.3d 605, 611 (7th Cir. 2000))

15. Elliott v. Jones, 2009 U.S. Dist. LEXIS 91125 (N.D. Fla. September 1, 2009)

16. Thompson v. Upshur County, 245 F.3d 447 (5th Cir. 2001)

17. Petties v. Carter, 836 F.3d 722, 728 (7th Cir. 2016) (en banc)

18. Gordon v. Cnty. of Orange, 888 F.3d 1118 (9th Cir. 2018)

19. Castro v. Cnty. of L.A., 833 F.3d 1060 (9th Cir. 2016)

20. Pittman by & through Hamilton v. County of Madison, Illinois 970 F.3d 823 (7th Cir. 2020)

21. Daniels v. Williams, 474 U.S. 327 (1986)

22. Hare v. City of Corinth, 74 F.3d 633 (5th Cir. 1996)

23. Estate of Cole v. Fromm, 94 F.3d 254 (7th Cir. 1996)

24. Palakovic v. Wetzel, 854 F.3d 209 (3d Cir. 2017)

25. Estate of Kempf v. Washington City, No. CV.15-1125,2018 WL4354547)

26. Lewis v. Cnty. of Northumberland, CIVIL ACTION No. 4:14-CV-02126, at *2 (M.D. Pa. December 15, 2016)

27. Williams, CJ. *Fault and the Suicide Victim: When Third Parties Assume a Suicide Victim's Duty of Self-Care.* 76 Neb. L. Rev. (1997)

28. Smith v. Jenkins, 919 F.2d 90 (8th Cir. 1990)

29. Monell v. New York City Dept. of Social Services, 436 U.S. 658 (1978)

30. Dixon v. Cnty. of Cook, 819 F.3d 343 (7th Cir. 2016)

31. Gable v. City of Chicago, 296 F.3d 531 (7th Cir. 2002)

32. Sims v. Mulcahy, 902 F.2d 524, 543 (7th Cir. 1990)

33. White v. Watson, No. 16-cv-560-JPG-DGW (S.D. Ill. Oct. 26, 2016)

34. Thomas v. Cook Cty Sheriff's Dept, 604 F.3d 293 (7th Cir. 2009)

35. Woodward v. Correctional Medical Services, 368 F.3d 917 (7th Cir. 2004)

36. Canton v. Harris, 489 U.S. 378 (1989)

37. Sornberger v. City of Knoxville, 434 F.3d 1006 (7th Cir. 2006)

38. Flores v. City of S. Bend, 997 F.3d 725 (7th Cir. 2021)

39. Harlow v. Fitzgerald, 457 U.S. 800 (1982)

40. Saucier v. Katz, 533 U.S. 194 (2001)

41. Mitchell v. Forsyth, 472 U.S. 511 (1985)

42. McNair v. Coffey, 279 F.3d 463 (7th Cir. 2002)

43. West v. Atkins, 487 U.S. 42 (1988)

44. Barnett v. Cnty. of Los Angeles, No. 2:20-cv-02530-ODW (ASx) (C.D. Cal. Sep. 3, 2020)

45. Jones v. Speidell, No. 1:16-cv-01335-DAD-SKO (P.C.), at *14 (E.D. Cal. May 15, 2017)

46. Bearden v. McKeithen, No. 5:11-cv-316-RS-EMT, at *13–14 (N.D. Fla. September 10, 2012)

47. A.H. v. St. Louis County Missouri, 891 F.3d 721, 729–39 (8th Cir. 2018)

48. Bryant v. Madigan, 84 F.3d 246, 249 (7th Cir. 1996)

49. Cox v. Callaway Cnty., No. 2:18-cv-04045-NKL (W.D. Mo. May 21, 2020)

50. Meagley v. City of Little Rock, 639 F.3d 384 (8th Cir. 2011)

51. Smith v. Harris Cnty., 956 F.3d 311 (5th Cir. 2020)

52. Smizer v. Standard, 16-CV-1476 (C.D. Ill. Jan. 20, 2017)

53. Trevino v. Woodbury Cnty. Jail, 623 F. App'x 824 (8th Cir. 2015)

54. Arenas v. Ga. Dep't of Corr., No. CV416-320 (S.D. Ga. Feb. 20, 2018)

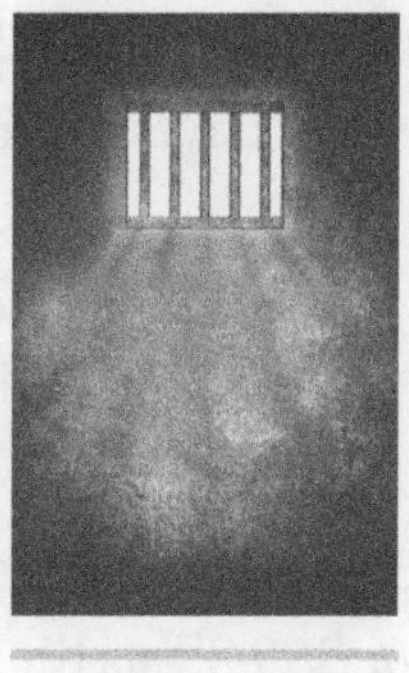

CHAPTER 7

LEGAL LIABILITY RISK MANAGEMENT

In jails and prisons, risk management has a dual emphasis: 1) Clinical management that is directed at reducing or eliminating inmate suicide and serious suicide attempts; and 2) avoiding legal liability. Clinical suicide risk management comprises ongoing identification of potential problems, suicide risk assessment, evidence-based best clinical and correctional practices, implementation of suicide prevention policies, procedure, and practice, and direct intervention and monitoring of inmates at risk (Chapters 2 to 5).

Adequate and consistent clinical risk management largely should eliminate legal liability in a typical inpatient or outpatient mental health setting. However, in a correctional setting, constitutional requirements of medical care, to some extent, determine risk management strategies and practice

(Chapter 6). In developing legal liability risk management strategies, court decisions have provided valuable insights and guidance.

In 2010, Darrell L. Ross, PhD, professor and the director of the School of Law Enforcement and Justice Administration at Western Illinois University, comprehensively reviewed 2,079 published §1983 court decisions from 1980 to 2008[1] with *Farmer v. Brennan* (1994)[2] as the midpoint to assess the impact of the Farmer decision. Jails comprised 75% (N. 1558) of the litigation, lockups 16% (N.336), and prisons 9% (N.185).

During the pre-*Farmer* period, correctional officials prevailed at the 3:1 ratio. Still, the ratio dropped to 4:1 post-*Farmer*, showing that the *Farmer* standard posed a higher hurdle to overcome for plaintiffs.

Ross cited policy violations, including failure to train the staff in 50% of the cases, medical/psychiatric care issues in 54%, and failure to protect in 55%. Multiple claims were common. Failing to protect, often targeted at correctional personnel, included failure to recognize suicidal ideation that was so obvious as to be recognizable to a layperson; failure to implement measures to reduce self-harm to the inmate; failure to recognize behaviors that may be associated with suicide; and failure to recognize an inmate's suicidal tendencies or past suicide attempts. Global issues included the agency failing to provide an adequate health-care system.

Lawsuits targeted health-care professionals, claiming they ignored, denied, or delayed medical care when such care was obvious. They also focused on the failure to assess the inmate at intake or the denial of access to health care and failure to provide adequate care during confinement.

COURT DECISIONS RELEVANT TO RISK MANAGEMENT
During the last forty years, courts have attempted to address issues about legal liability related to suicide. The decisions cover various situations in jails and prisons, including diagnosis, monitoring, treatment, communication, policies, staffing, and training.

Historically, whether an inmate has received adequate medical care has been viewed through the lens of the Eighth Amendment, which prohibits cruel and unusual punishment. Such cases require a showing of deliberate indifference, and it is primarily those cases that are discussed here. However, inmates who are in jail awaiting trial (called pretrial detainees), cannot be subject to any punishment. There is a growing movement among courts to analyze such cases under the Fourth Amendment, which prohibits unreasonable seizures. In such a case, a plaintiff would not have to prove deliberate indifference, only that the care he or she received was not reasonable under the circumstances (*Miranda v. County of Lake*).[3]

1. *Inadequacy of mental health evaluation*
In *Comstock v. McCrary*[4] psychologist Norris McCrary did not perform an adequate psychological evaluation and risk assessment the day Billy Wade Montgomery (decedent) committed suicide. The psychologist took the decedent's denial of suicide ideation and plan at face value, although he knew Montgomery had been a suicide risk a day earlier and had placed him on suicide watch. Had McCrary done a detailed psychological evaluation, he would have known that the decedent was feeling beset by several enemies that called him a snitch.

A casual and cursory mental health or psychiatric evaluation of inmates who conceal their true intent may result in legal liability claims.

2. *Failure to identify obvious and substantial risk factors*

In ***Williams v. Mehra***[5] the significant issue involved a failure to identify an inmate's obvious and substantial suicide risk factors that included depression, psychiatric hospitalization, suicide ideation, and a previous suicide attempt with antidepressant tablets.

During pretrial detention in the Wayne County Jail, lasting about sixteen months from April 1992 to August 1993, Anthony Wade was diagnosed with clinical depression with psychotic features and suicidal thoughts. He was treated with Thorazine. In December 1992, he attempted suicide, overdosing with 20 tablets of Thorazine 50 mg, which he'd hoarded from his pill line. Due to the deterioration of his condition, he was transferred to a psychiatric hospital on February 18, 1993. The prognosis was noted as "guarded" due to his noncompliance. A psychiatrist at the hospital prescribed liquid Sinequan to manage his depression. Upon return to jail, Wade was maintained on the same liquid medication. During the final interview at the jail, before he was transferred to a prison to serve his sentence, Wade reported continuing thoughts of suicide. He had a suicide plan, which he refused to share with anyone. This information was noted in the jail discharge form that also indicated his diagnosis of depression, treatment with liquid Sinequan, and the fact that he had a suicide plan but refused to share it with a therapist or correctional officers.

A prison psychiatrist prescribed Sinequan tablets instead of the liquid form, despite the information in the discharge form. However, this psychiatrist did not review the discharge form. During his monthly scheduled psychiatric follow-up, another psychiatrist determined that Wade was depressed but not at suicide risk because he denied suicidal ideation. He increased the dose of Sinequan tablets and added Ascendin, another antidepressant in tablet form. Wade was then transferred to a different cell block where he was seen by another psychiatrist, who determined that he was depressed and had some suicidal ideation. On August 18, 1993, a psychologist who saw him thought that he was ambivalent about killing himself. Five days later, Wade took his life with Sinequan tablets he hoarded from the pill line.

Besides failure to identify the obvious and substantial risk factors, the psychiatrists neglected to review the discharge form that contained Wade's diagnosis, suicidality, and specific treatment measure to address his suicidality, (i.e., prescribing liquid medication). Also, procedurally, the nursing staff, who dispensed his medication on the pill line, failed to manage his psychiatric medication intake on a watch-take basis.

3. *Issues related to psychotropic medication practice*

In *Greason v. Kemp*[6] the court held that abrupt discontinuation of psychotropic medications of an inmate with a recent history of suicide attempt constituted deliberate indifference. Charles Greason, a Georgia prison inmate, killed himself while incarcerated. The plaintiffs claimed that the decedent committed suicide because the defendants—the prison officials responsible for his custody and those who provided his mental health care—were deliberately indifferent to his psychiatric needs.

The doctor had abruptly discontinued Greason's antidepressant medication without reviewing his clinical file, conducting a mental status examination, or ordering close monitoring. In this case, other issues identified by the court included the doctor's failure to review his medical files, the department's failure to train the staff, inadequate mental health care delivery, and delayed or denied treatment.

In *Steele v. Shah*[7] a psychiatrist at Polk Correctional Institution diagnosed William Steele with adjustment disorder with depressed mood, and he prescribed Prozac and Tofranil. Steele had a long history of drug addiction and had attempted suicide twice before starting his twenty-five-year sentence. When he entered prison, he was facing divorce from his wife of fourteen years. A psychologist found him emotionally labile. Although Steele gradually improved, he became anxious just before he was transferred to another facility, the Orange County Jail. He arrived at the new facility with a discharge note that he should be referred to a psychiatrist. Five days later, in an interview that lasted less than a minute, Dr. Mahendra Shah at Orange County Jail told Steele that his medications would be discontinued. Steele asked Dr. Shah to explain why Shah was discontinuing the medications. Dr. Shah stated, "You are dismissed."

Steele experienced intense anxiety, insomnia, and physical pain. He contacted providers at his former institution and wrote two letters showing his helplessness and hopelessness. A nurse reached out to the medical staff supervisor at Orange County jail and informed her that Steele was a suicide risk, and had been aggressively treated with Prozac and Tofranil. The psychiatrist at his former prison followed up with a letter detailing Steele's condition and reiterating that he was a suicide risk. Steele remained without medication for 182 days at Orange County Jail. As soon as he reached his former institution, he was restarted on his medications.

Steele filed a suit claiming deliberate indifference for 1) discontinuing his medication without examining him; 2) the psychiatrist at Orange County jail not reviewing his medical records; and 3) not consulting his former providers.

The district court granted Dr. Shah's motion for a summary judgment, indicating that his decision was nothing more than a disputed medical opinion. On appeal, the Eleventh Circuit held that "psychiatric needs can constitute serious medical needs and that the quality of psychiatric care one receives can be so substantial a deviation from the accepted standards as to evidence deliberate indifference to those serious psychiatric needs." Citing *Greason v. Kemp*,[6] the court opined "there exists a clearly established right to have (one's) psychotropic medication continued if discontinuation would amount to grossly inadequate psychiatric care."

One district court held that the failure of the jail's nursing staff to investigate what medication an inmate was taking immediately prior to his admission could constitute deliberate indifference.

When Ryan Clark (*Estate of Ryan Clark v. County of Green Lake*)[8] was admitted to jail in a highly intoxicated state, he told the intake officer and the jail nurse that he had been taking anti-depressant medication but could not remember its name. The nurse did not obtain Clark's signature on a consent form to contact his parents or the pharmacy to learn about what medications he had been taking, did not contact the jail's on-call physician, and made no attempt to learn which medication he had been taking so the medication could be continued. Her motion for summary judgment was denied. The court noted that the nurse knew Clark from previous incarcerations, knew he had suffered from chronic depression, knew he was at greater risk of suicide due to his state of intoxication, and that she may have disregarded "red flags" regarding his mental health.

4. *Officers' failure to communicate an arrestee's suicide statements*

In **Gordon v. Kidd**[9] the court established that failure by an arresting officer to communicate relevant information to booking officers can constitute deliberate indifference. Officer Gordon Lyman filled out a police report of the arrest of Clarence Gordon that included a statement that "the suspect's wife said that the suspect was going to kill himself."

Officer Lyman passed the custody of Gordon to Officer John Smith, assistant supervisor of the jail because Lyman was scheduled to leave his shift. Though Smith initially denied hearing anything about Gordon's statement, he later admitted that Lyman told him: "He may try to hang himself. Here is his belt."

Smith said Lyman also warned him that "you'd better watch this fellow." Smith claimed he did not take Lyman's warning seriously because Lyman's manner did not convey that Gordon was serious, even though Lyman admitted that Gordon could easily have done so [committed suicide]. Officer Smith told no one in the jail of Lyman's warning. He not only failed to make a note of the information he received from Lyman, but also he did not request the jail nurse to perform a suicide screening of Gordon for suicidal tendencies, as jail policy required. He ignored the information Lyman gave him and passed Gordon on to other officers without transmitting Lyman's statement. Gordon was placed in a holding cell. During an interview with a medical nurse, he admitted to two heart attacks and treatment for depression. Because Gordon became combative, the nurse was unable to complete the medical screening. Gordon was found dead a few hours later. Lyman's warning to Officer Smith constituted sufficient notice that Gordon's suicide attempt might be imminent.

Smith's request for summary judgment was denied, because he knew of Gordon's imminent suicide risk, and was deliberately indifferent to that risk. On appeal, the appellate court opined that "Smith's failure to take any action in response to the information he received sustains the district court's denial of his motion for summary judgment."

In *Freedman v. City of Allentown*[10] in contrast to *Gordon v. Kidd*[9] and *Conn v. City of Reno*,[11] a probation officer, Frank Koboth, *had* knowledge of an arrestee's past suicide attempt, but the court decided that his failure did not reach the threshold of deliberate indifference when he failed to inform the arresting officer. The allegations against Kroboth included the information that Kroboth, who knew of Jerry Freedman's prior suicide attempt, failed to inform Officer Carl Balliet, who was then questioning Freedman, of Freedman's suicidal tendencies. A reasonably prudent probation officer, knowing that Freedman was being questioned or had been detained, would have cautioned the detaining officers about Freedman's prior suicide attempt and suicidal tendencies. The court noted that "At most the averments against Kroboth amount to a lack of due care and are not actionable as a §1983 claim."

5. *Suicidal ideation, suicide watch, and logging*

Management of inmates who deny suicidal ideation is a complex issue because mental health professionals often release inmates who deny suicidal ideation from suicide watch. It is well established in psychiatric literature that some inmates intentionally conceal their true intent after they make their decision to exit the world.

Failure to institute suicide watch if the evaluator considers the inmate statements as non-serious, manipulative, and lacking intent is another complicating issue. Premature discontinuation of suicide watch, ordered without an adequate suicide risk assessment, gives the opportunity for a suicidal inmate to take his life.

In *Woodward v. Myres*, discussed in Chapter 4, the claims centered on the failure to institute standard suicide watch, lack of suicide watch monitoring and logging, abrupt and premature discontinuation of suicide watch, and noncompliance with the facility's suicide prevention, policies, and practice.

In *Simmons v. Navajo County*[12] the court opined that placing a pretrial detainee on suicide watch, even the highest level, standing alone "does not demonstrate that an official was subjectively aware of a substantial risk of imminent suicide." However, in day-to-day correctional practice, inmates' history of placement on suicide watch is considered an indicator of suicidal propensity. As per Simmons' court, determinants of imminent suicide risk include "observed suicidal actions, heard statements of a suicidal nature, or witnessed other evidence of decedent's suicidal intent" that would have alerted the official that the inmate has an impending suicidal crisis.

In *Hott v. Minnesota*, discussed in Chapter 6, falsification of suicide watch by an officer resulted in an unfavorable court decision for the officer. Falsification of a suicide watch log, not an uncommon occurrence, almost always results in settlement of the case.

In *Minix v. Canarecci*[13] the district court opined that there was enough evidence to allow a jury to find a direct causal link between the jail's practice of classifying and releasing detainees from suicide watch and Gregory Zick's suicide.

Zick was booked at the St. Joseph County Jail on March 22, 2003. The booking officer noted that Zick had self-inflicted scars on his arms and neck, had suicidal thoughts, a history of psychiatric hospitalization, and had attempted suicide a month before. During his initial classification and booking, Zick told an officer that he "planned" his suicide attempts. He stated that he was taking medications including Paxil, Depakote, and Buspar, and his mother confirmed his medications. After an evaluation by the medical staff, he was placed in the medical segregation unit. Two days later, Nurse Jeanne James recommended moving him to the general population because he "no longer needed medical observation; denied suicidal tendencies."

Zick was placed in medical segregation again on suicide watch on April 21, 2003, because he refused his medication and was thought to be suicidal. Again, Nurse James removed him from suicide watch and transferred him out of medical segregation. Shortly after the second transfer, he hanged himself in his cell.

Cathy Minix, Zink's mother, filed a lawsuit against Nurse James and Dr. David, the jail's medical director, claiming deliberate indifference in discontinuing Zick's suicide watch on April 23, 2003, and transferring him to the general population.

Dr. David took the position that he "didn't have control as far as saying [Gregory] needed to be in suicide watch or he didn't need to be in suicide watch." Nurse James did not believe he was an imminent suicide risk because he denied suicidal ideation. Therefore, Nurse James did not contact Dr. David (or any other physician) before deciding to transfer Zick out of suicide watch on April 23, 2003.

The Seventh Circuit held that although the decision to release Zick from medical observation might, in hindsight, be seen to have been a mistake; that James did not act with deliberate indifference to a known risk that Zick would take his own life. Before his final release from medical segregation in April 2003, Zick had been under observation for two days, during which time he denied suicidal thoughts. He displayed similar behavior shortly before his release from the first suicide watch. The court noted, "Given Gregory's denials of suicide, James had no actual knowledge that Gregory would imminently seek to take his own life."

Dr. David, the director of medical services, was not directly involved in Zick's treatment except to approve the prescription medications that he received at the jail. The Seventh Circuit found this lack of direct participation made Minix's individual-capacity claim against David more difficult, since individual liability under §1983 requires "personal involvement in the alleged constitutional deprivation. To be personally liable under these circumstances, David must have condoned or acquiesced in a subordinate's decision." In *Minix*, the court found the medical director not liable for the nurse's alleged deliberate indifference because there was no evidence suggesting the director condoned such practices. Furthermore, the medical director's non-involvement did not amount to deliberate indifference.

In ***Broughton v. Premier Health Care Services***[14] the issue was intentional concealment of suicidal ideation that made it difficult to stake a successful claim of deliberate indifference against correctional officials.

The Sixth Circuit affirmed the district court granting summary judgment for the officers who were alleged to have violated Steven Broughton's Eighth Amendment protection. Broughton was booked in Warren County Jail on June 24, 2011. The medical screening form completed by a correctional officer showed that Broughton told the officer he was not having suicidal thoughts, and had last attempted suicide three years ago. However, nine days earlier, he had been hospitalized for an attempted overdose. He had tried to overdose on drugs "[o]ver a dozen" times since he was nine years old. None of this, however, was known to the medical staff at Warren County Jail. In fact, Broughton intentionally concealed his history of mental illness and attempted suicide because, in his words, he "didn't want to be placed on suicide watch."

Broughton was ultimately admitted to the general population and, after getting into an argument with his cellmate, was placed in disciplinary segregation without any suicide prevention protocols. About a day and a half later, on July 1, 2011, he attempted to kill himself while alone in his cell. The correctional officers discovered him hanging by a sheet. They cut him down, resuscitated him, and transported him to a hospital, where he recovered.

The court opined, "While Broughton's disclaimer of suicidal ideation does not automatically insulate the defendants from liability, it does undermine the claim that they willfully ignored his past medical history and current symptomology."

Strickler v. Mc Cord[15] illustrates the difficulty for jail personnel charged with the care of inmates who are determined to commit suicide. Because Donald Strickler was serious about ending his life, he deliberately hid his intentions from anyone who might have been able to prevent it. After his arrest following a car accident, he was sent to Bowen Center for evaluation for attempted suicide, as it was his second attempt. He denied that the car accident was a suicide attempt, claiming that he blacked out due to intoxication and hit a tree.

At the Bowen Center, Strickler told the staff that he was suicidal because he "didn't want to get locked up in an insane asylum." When asked about suicidal thoughts or a plan to commit suicide, he responded, "Not today." He was then sent to Miami County Jail, where he answered "no" to questions designed to elicit suicide ideation and behaviors. His wife and mother expressed concern that he might be suicidal.

However, the officers kept him in line of sight in a glass cell. A counselor interviewed Strickler. In his report, under the heading "Presenting problem and history," the counselor noted, "suicidal thoughts [continue], his wife is divorcing him, and he does not feel he has much to live for." Under danger to self, he checked yes for "thoughts of suicide," and "threats of suicide," but not for "suicide plan," "suicide attempts," "preoccupation with death," "suicide gesture," or "family history of suicide." It also noted that Strickler had not been able to find work for several months. The counselor diagnosed him with alcohol dependence and depression and recommended that Strickler be put in the general jail population. Officers tried to put him on suicide watch, but he denied suicidal ideation. A substance abuse evaluation showed that he was at moderate self-harm risk. Shortly after this interview, he began hiding his Prozac. However, officers did not know about it. He pried out blades from razors, and he concealed them from officers.

The court found that "He lied on the intake form; he lied when questioned about suicidal thoughts at the Bowen Center, and he deceived the guards about his medication and the razor blades." The court opined in granting a summary judgment for the defendants that his "suicide attempt was tragic, but the facts of this case, taken as a whole, do not support even an inference that the defendants had actual knowledge of a substantial risk that Strickler was serious about killing himself."

6. *Recent Suicide Attempt and Failure To Get Prior Medical Records*

A recent suicide attempt is the most significant predictor of suicide. The courts have not opined on the recency of suicide attempt relevant to a liability claim. Clinically, a near-lethal suicide attempt within six months to a year has a higher likelihood of a future completed suicide. Although past suicide attempt is not predictive, it increases lifetime suicide vulnerability.

From a legal perspective, failure to question an inmate about a history of past suicide attempts can lead to potential liability.

While some inmates intentionally withhold the information, the prior records serve as the most reliable vehicle to get such information. One way to prevail in a lawsuit against corrections officials is for a plaintiff to establish that the decedent previously made near-lethal suicide attempt/s or had history of a pattern of suicidal behavior. Prison officials must make a reasonable effort to gather at-risk inmate's history of prior suicide attempts or a pattern of suicidal behaviors.

In *Terry v. Rice*[16] county officials went out of their way not to collect information from the prison where the decedent was transferred presumably for "safekeeping." On March 21, 1998, about three weeks before he killed himself, Sheriff Rice at Montgomery County Jail transferred Donald Terry to the Indiana Department of Correction's Reception and Diagnostic Center (RDC), after Terry cut himself on his wrist, causing a deep laceration and after he injured another inmate. During his six-day stay at the RDC from March 21 to 27, 1998, an RDC psychiatrist determined Terry as a suicide threat, because he made suicidal statements. The psychiatrist put Terry on a suicide watch and increased Terry's dose of Thorazine from 50 mg to 150 mg a day. However, Sheriff Rice got him transferred back to the jail after six days—ostensibly for cost-saving. Terry had a long-standing history of mental illness with paranoid schizophrenia and suicide attempts during his multiple incarcerations at Montgomery County Jail. Upon transfer back to the jail, neither the sheriff, deputy sheriff, nor the jail nurse ever inquired about Terry's stay at RDC or asked for any medical records. The court found Sheriff Rice deliberately chose not to find out how RDC staff had handled Terry for purposes of "safekeeping," at Sheriff Rice's "own request."

In denying the motion for summary judgment, the court opined that "Going out of your way to avoid acquiring unwelcome knowledge is a species of intent. Being an ostrich involves a level of knowledge sufficient for conviction of crimes requiring specific intent," citing *Comstock v. McCrary,* where Norris McCrary, a psychologist, presumably did not want to know about the inmate's special circumstances of being called a snitch by his enemies.

In *McKee v. Turner*[17] the treating psychiatrist was sued for failing to get prior jail records that indicated the decedent had attempted suicide by hanging six weeks before he arrived at the prison. The dissenting judge felt the facts did not support the claim of deliberate indifference. However, the dissenting judge opined, "McKee is distinguishable in one specific aspect, (i.e., failure to obtain medical records)" in that consulting prior mental health records of an inmate with a history of recent suicide attempt is a standard procedure to determine the current risk. The psychiatrist was aware of the decedent's previous suicide attempt but failed to get his prior records. Plaintiff presented the affidavit of an opposing psychiatrist who stated that "he would have discovered information about the decedent's suicidal tendencies if the treating psychiatrist had obtained the medical records."

7. *Diagnosis and Treatment Issues*

Prisoners have claimed several diagnostic and treatment issues to support §1983 claims.

a) *Diagnosis of mental illness*

The diagnosis of a mental disorder or failure to diagnose per se does not support a claim of deliberate indifference liability. While inmates with the diagnosis of depression, anxiety, and bipolar disorder have a high degree of suicidal propensity, unless indicators of suicide vulnerability accompany the diagnosis, the claim is not sustainable.

Some inmates, including those with antisocial personality disorder, display erratic and strange behaviors such as responding to hallucinations, smearing feces on cell walls, flooding the cell, "eating blades," and other strange behaviors. These behaviors may be symptoms of serious mental illness but not necessarily indications of suicidal risk. The courts have held that displays of erratic behavior or signs of mental illness, without specific indicia of suicidal tendency, "do not rise to the level of a strong risk of suicide" and do not provide "the level of notice" required to trigger the deliberate indifference standard. In *Jackson v. West*[18] the Eleventh Circuit court found that corrections officers did not subjectively appreciate a strong likelihood of suicide because of either the inmate's antisocial and aggressive behavior, or his verbal suicide threats months before his actual suicide, when medical staff had addressed those threats and cleared the inmate to return to the general population.

In *Cavalieri v. Shepard*[19] quoting *Estate of Novack v. County of Wood*[20] the Seventh Circuit has said that "strange behavior alone, without indications that that behavior has a substantial likelihood of taking a suicidal turn, is not sufficient to impute subjective knowledge of a high suicide risk to jail personnel." But odd behavior coupled with actual information that the individual is at risk of suicide can be sufficient to infer awareness on the part of a defendant. In *Cavalieri*, the court further stated, "Indeed, had no one informed (officer) Shepard that Steven was at risk of suicide, this would be a different case. But both Mrs. Cavalieri (mother) and Rouse (girlfriend) testified that they had alerted Shepard to this specific risk. Shepard was not forced to operate only based on a brief observation."

b) *Incorrect diagnosis*

In *Steele v. Choi*[21] the court concluded incorrect diagnosis or improper treatment does not support an Eighth Amendment claim. In affirming a summary judgment in favor of Dr. Choi, the Seventh Circuit opined that "*Estelle* requires us to distinguish between 'deliberate indifference' to serious medical needs of prisoners on the one hand, and 'negligence' in diagnosing or treating a medical condition." Dr. Choi misdiagnosed Steele's symptoms as Percocet overdose despite the absence of evidence of such a diagnosis. His condition later turned out to be subarachnoid hemorrhage from a ruptured aneurysm, which was surgically repaired. However, Steele suffered significantly. The court emphasized that malpractice is not enough proof under *Farmer*. Furthermore, "Some other medical professional would have chosen a different course of treatment was also insufficient to establish a constitutional deliberate indifference claim." Incorrect diagnosis may support a claim of medical malpractice but not a claim of deliberate indifference. Again, what is required is the indicia of suicide risk.

c) *Intentional refusal to provide medical care*

Courts have acknowledged that intentionally refusing to respond to an inmate's complaints, including repeated requests to see a mental health professional or physician, may constitute deliberate indifference. To prevail, the plaintiff must establish that the providers intentionally refused to provide medical care or denied access to a physician, and that such refusal must cause the inmate undue suffering or threat of injury. Often in jails and prisons, the care is prompt and timely compared with care rendered in the outside community. Therefore, the key element that supports a deliberate indifference claim is willful refusal of services.

d) *Delays in treatment*

Courts have established that repeated delays in treatment of medical or dental conditions were sufficient to state a claim of deliberate medical indifference.[22, 23] The conditions must be sufficiently serious, causing pain, infection, and functional limitations such as the inability to eat, but not necessarily be life-threatening. However, isolated delays or delays due to the natural course of events in a facility and administrative procedures, not an uncommon occurrence in a correctional setting, may not be actionable.

Meritorious claims of delay of treatment depend on the length of delay, the nature of the medical need, and the reason for the delay.[18] In *Harris v. Coweta County*[24] Harris suffered a "prominent and unexplained" two-month delay in treatment for a painful hand condition. The court held, "Delay in treatment of serious and painful injuries was also clearly recognized as rising to the level of a constitutional claim."

Delaying treatment may constitute deliberate indifference if such delay exacerbated the injury or unnecessarily prolonged an inmate's pain."[25, 26, 27] However, the Eighth Amendment does not give prisoners entitlement to "demand specific care" or "the best care possible," but requires only "reasonable measures to meet a substantial risk of serious harm."[28] Courts know that jails and prisons have limited resources and take that factor into consideration in decision-making.

Delay in responding to repeated requests to see a mental health professional by an inmate who is potentially suicidal may be effectively claimed by a plaintiff. In *Quinn v. Lashbrook*[29] the court decided a claim of delayed treatment was meritorious. The courts generally dismiss any claims that are considered frivolous or malicious. A mental health professional assessed Chester O'Quinn as a suicide risk and placed him on suicide watch but not in a health care unit, as O'Quinn wanted. Instead, he was placed in a segregation cell, almost naked in unsanitary conditions. He was denied showers. Despite his repeated complaints to the officers and the warden, and grievances about the deplorable conditions, his pleas were ignored.

Plaintiff (O'Quinn) alleged that he put in several sick-call requests upon his release from suicide watch, which the mental health professionals ignored, causing him to become more depressed. The court found O'Quinn had sufficiently stated an Eighth Amendment deliberate indifference claim against the defendants, including officers and mental health professionals, to support a claim based on delayed treatment to proceed.

It is true that delays in care for "non-life-threatening but painful conditions may constitute deliberate indifference if the delay exacerbated the injury or unnecessarily prolonged an inmate's pain." Yet prisons have limited resources, and that fact makes some delay inevitable. For a delay in treatment to qualify as deliberate indifference, we must weigh "the seriousness of the condition and the ease of providing treatment" (*Mitchell v. Kallas*).[30] (Internal quotations and citations omitted)

Failing to provide care for a non-medical reason, if that care has been recommended by a medical specialist, can constitute deliberate indifference.[27] Continuing treatment that has proven to be ineffective can also constitute deliberate indifference. The Seventh Circuit opined in *Goodloe v. Sood*[25] citing *Greeno v. Daley*[31]: "Put most bluntly, faced with an inmate experiencing ongoing suffering from a serious medical condition, a prison physician cannot 'doggedly persis[t] in a course of treatment known to be ineffective' without violating the Eighth Amendment."

e) *Improper medication or modality of treatment*

Improper medication treatment and medical supervision by the psychiatrist can support a claim of deliberate indifference if it can be proved such improper medication treatment cause suicidal ideation and serious injury resulting in death. Prisoners are not entitled to a specific prescription or modality of treatment if the choice of medication prescribed by the physician, or the modality of treatment does address his medical need.

Failing to provide care for a non-medical reason, if that care has been recommended by a medical specialist, can constitute deliberate indifference.[27]

f) *Inadequate treatment and difference in medical decisions*

In ***Durmer v. O'Carroll***[32] the court opined that not all inadequate treatment provided to a prisoner can be construed as deliberately indifferent. It can simply be "no more than mere negligence." The court further opined that if inadequate treatment results simply from an error in medical judgment, there is no constitutional violation. The Durmer court added that a non-physician defendant cannot be considered deliberately indifferent for failing to respond to an inmate's medical complaints when he is already receiving treatment by the prison's medical staff. Furthermore, the court held that prison administrators cannot be deliberately indifferent "simply because they failed to respond directly to the medical complaints of a prisoner who was already being treated by the prison doctor." However, where a failure or delay in providing prescribed treatment is deliberate and motivated by non-medical factors, a constitutional claim may be presented.[33]

In ***Arenas v. GA Department Corrections et al.***[34] the court found a failure to provide adequate treatment to young Richard Tavera, who had a long-standing history of depression and bipolar disorder. In 2014 at age twenty-four, he committed suicide at Smith State Prison. Tavera had attempted suicide at age sixteen and, as a result, was hospitalized. After this hospitalization, Tavera was prescribed medication to treat his bipolar disorder.

In ***Norfleet v. Webster***[35] the court noted that "A difference of opinion among physicians on how an inmate should be treated will not support a finding of deliberate indifference." Evidence that some medical professionals would have chosen a different course of treatment than what an inmate received or requested is insufficient to make out a constitutional claim.[21]

To be able to prove deliberate indifference based on the treatment decision of a doctor or nurse, that treatment must have been so far afield of accepted professional standards as to raise the inference that the decision to go forward with that treatment was not based on medical judgment.[36]

g) *Inadequate monitoring of inmates in administrative segregation*

Periodic reviews of an inmate's suitability to continued stay in administrative segregation is a standard procedure. Courts have recognized "substantial risk of psychological harm and decompensation posed by extended placement in segregation" including anxiety, panic, paranoia, depression, PTSD, psychosis, and disintegration of basic sense of self-identity.[37] Substantial harm can result from "inadequate periodic mental-health evaluations in segregation" as reflected in the "high numbers of suicide deaths, and incidents of self-harm and self-mutilation that occur in many of these units."[38]

h) *Intoxicated detainees*

In *Frey v. Herculaneum*[39] a claim of deliberate indifference was filed by the father of Arthur Frey Jr., who was arrested by City of Herculaneum police for driving while intoxicated. He hanged himself with a bedsheet in Pevely Jail several hours later. Frey's father alleged that the Herculaneum police "(1) were deliberately indifferent to the medical needs of Frey insofar as they knew or should have known he was a suicide risk; (2) knew or should have known he was in need of immediate medical attention; (3) inadequately monitored the jail cells; (4) failed to take precautions to remove dangerous items from Frey's cell; and (5) knew or should have known that the jail was defective and dangerous." The district court granted the city's motions to dismiss for failure to state a cause of action. On appeal, the Eighth Circuit reversed and remanded to the district court with directions for the court to allow Frey to amend his complaint.

The court considered a proposed amended complaint in which specific allegations were made against individual officers who knew or should have known that Frey talked about suicide, put a gun in his mouth, had a severe drug and alcohol problem, and admitted being ill. Moreover, an officer knew or should have known that Frey had threatened to kill both himself and his wife during the previous month.

i) *Policy, staffing, and training*

In many deliberate indifference lawsuits, counties face Monell claims related to suicide prevention policy, mental health and correctional staffing, and training.

1. *Absence of suicide prevention policy*

Absence of suicide prevention policy would create a situation where the necessary procedures and practice supporting risk identification, assessment, and monitoring could not be effectively carried out, causing risk of harm to inmates.

Absence of a suicide prevention policy per se does not prevent officials from responding appropriately to suicide threat: they can properly respond—and do—in the absence of a policy. But when they don't, the lack of an adequate policy strengthens a deliberate indifference claim against the municipality (county), since the failure to properly respond to the threat of suicide is exactly what a suicide policy is designed to prevent. Still, though, courts properly applying the deliberate indifference standard would have to determine that the policymakers who failed to adopt a suicide prevention policy did so with deliberate indifference to the need to adopt such a policy. In other words, the officials would have to know that the very lack of a policy was creating a substantial risk of death and serious bodily injury.

In *White v. Watson*[40] Bradley C. Scarpi, a pretrial detainee in St. Clair County Jail from April 14, 2014, committed suicide in his cell on May 23, 2014. Scarpi suffered from mental illness and drug addiction. He had been incarcerated several times during the ten years before he took his life. On May 23, 2014, at 4:00 p.m., Scarpi was moved to a different cell due to his fear of enemies. When he complained of enemies in his new cell block, he was moved to maximum security block in a regular cell. On his way, he told the officers that he was going to kill himself. An officer in charge of him told him to be quiet and even dared him to go ahead. A fellow inmate told the officer that Scarpi would kill himself. Scarpi was not monitored or given any mental health services.

Scarpi's brother, his personal representative, filed a deliberate indifference lawsuit against County Sheriff Watson, on the basis that St. Clair County Jail did not have a suicide prevention policy, did not provide adequate training and supervision of employees on suicide prevention, and had a practice of routinely denying mentally ill detainees access to mental health services and suicide-proof cells. To support that the sheriff was aware of Scarpi's risk, the plaintiff presented data showing two suicides and fourteen suicide attempts in the jail between January 2014 and October 2015.

The court opined that the absence of suicide prevention policy and lack of training and supervision were "the moving force behind the failure to protect Scarpi from the known risk of suicide in the Jail. This is sufficient to state a §1983 claim under Monell for deliberate indifference to a detainee's safety needs."

The Supreme Court has expressly acknowledged that evidence of a single violation of federal rights can trigger municipal liability if the violation was a "highly predictable consequence" of the municipality's failure to act.[41]

In *Terry v. Rice*[16] the county did not have a policy to implement proper procedures for dealing with mentally ill or suicidal inmates or getting inmates' medical records from community sources.

In denying the summary judgment motion by Sheriff Rice, the court opined that "Where a municipality has failed to make a policy in a situation that calls for procedures, rules, or regulations, the failure itself might be actionable." It further noted the plaintiff must come forward with evidence not only of the case but also of a "pattern or series of incidents of unconstitutional conduct" or a failure to act knowing that the situation was certain to recur.[16] The active policy when the decedent took his life dealt only with inmates as they were booked into the jail and did not provide any kind of screening mechanism or address the needs of established inmates.

2. *Policy or custom causing or contributing risk of harm*

In **Gibson v. County of Washoe**[42] Stephen Gibson suffered a heart attack and died on February 3, 1996, while in the custody of the Washoe County, Nevada, Sheriff's Department. Gibson suffered from manic depressive disorder with a history of multiple hospitalizations since 1991 and was under the care of a psychiatrist who prescribed him medications to control his mania. At the time of arrest and booking, he displayed erratic and uncontrollable behaviors, for which he was placed in soft restraints. From 1995 until 1999, the jail did not have mental health workers to perform mental health screening. Consequently, the County did not screen detainees at the jail.

Ms. Gibson alleged that the County failed to train the deputies in recognizing signs of mental illness. In granting summary judgment, the district court opined that Gibson's serious medical condition caused his death, and the deputies were not deliberately indifferent to his mental illness.

The defendants' medical expert testified that Gibson's uncontrolled manic state and the officers' efforts to restrain him "resulted in a physiologically stressful state for Mr. Gibson, which essentially resulted in a heart attack."

The Ninth Circuit reversed the decision, concluding that "summary judgment was improperly granted on the question whether the County was deliberately indifferent to Gibson's mental illness while he was in custody at the county jail." The court opined that County's failure to respond to Gibson's urgent need for medical attention was a direct result of "an affirmative County policy that was deliberately indifferent, under the Farmer standard, to this need." Because Gibson was combative and uncooperative, no medical evaluation took place.

Multiple policies or practices that combine to deprive a prisoner of a "single, identifiable human need," such as mental health care, can support a finding of Eighth Amendment liability[43] (recognizing 'totality of conditions' approach in prison-conditions cases). [38]

3. *Shortage of staff*

In ***Bragg v. Dunn***[38] the court cited persistent and severe mental health and correctional staff shortages, combined with chronic and significant overcrowding, as the "overarching issues that permeate" the factors that contribute to inadequate mental health care. Shortage of mental health staff has a direct impact on the identification of mentally ill and suicidal inmates, monitoring and treating them.

4. *Failure to train*

Cases that allege failure to train the staff are based on the U.S. Supreme Court decision in ***City of Canton v. Harris***.[44] A county can be found deliberately indifferent if it fails to train officers to recognize suicide indicators, policy issues, monitoring procedures, and how to obtain medical or mental health care.

A court may reject a plaintiff's claims if the defendant can show evidence of training and/or policies that directed officers in responding to detainees who exhibit a "strong likelihood" of suicide. Officers cannot be held liable for deliberate indifference "unless an inmate was so obviously mentally ill that the deputies, who had received

> no training regarding the diagnosis and treatment of mental illness, must have known that [he] was exhibiting symptoms of mental illness."[12]

STRATEGIES TO AVOID LAWSUITS

Suicide prevention practices and court decisions must guide the stakeholders to develop legal liability risk management strategies at administrative, clinical, and custody/jail staff levels. The clinical, programmatic, and research-based strategies depend on legally defensible, clinically sound policies, procedures, and practices. Specifically, the policies must cover suicide prevention and intervention, delivery of mental health services, and medication administration, including involuntary medication and treatment of the seriously mentally ill. The mental health (MH) services delivery system must ensure inmates' access to mental health services. To that extent, timely response to Medical Services Request (MSR) would avoid any delay in mental health and psychiatric services, precluding any liability lawsuits claiming delay in services.

Correctional administrators must take the lead in establishing suicide prevention as an institutional priority, communicating the goal clearly and consistently to all staff, and providing the necessary resources. The administration must create an attitude among the staff that most suicides and serious suicide attempts are preventable.

Professional standards dictate that the duty of care includes three phases: assessment, treatment, and follow-up. The most significant component of duty of care regarding suicide risk is assessment. Assessment includes evaluation of an inmate's likelihood for self-injury with significant emphasis on risk factors including verbalization of suicidal thoughts, plans, behavior, and nonverbal cues of self-harm such as change in behaviors, giving away possessions, acute or chronic mental illness, prior serious attempt, substance abuse, acute psychosocial stressors including recent losses, trauma, and legal/parole setbacks as well as historical indicators.

Training employees on suicide prevention, policy, procedures, and practice, and mental illness is the most effective tool to prevent most suicides. Upon initial employment and on an ongoing basis, all correctional and mental health staff should be trained on all aspects of suicide prevention, including mental disorders and suicide-prevention policies, procedures, and practices.

CRITICAL PROCEDURES AND PRACTICE

The most critical procedures and practices to mitigate risk of legal action, based on court decisions include the following:

1. Timely communication by arresting officers to booking officers regarding
   a. Arrestee's behavior
   b. Arrestee's statements and emotional state
   c. Officer's impression of the arrestee's potential suicide risk
   d. Communication by spouse, family members, and those present at the scene
2. Suicide Screening
   a. Systematic and routine suicide screening with emphasis on current suicidal ideation, intent, and plan

    b. Past near-lethal suicide attempts and the time frame

    c. Obtaining medical records from community sources

3. Systematic, routine, and repeat suicide risk assessment of inmates at risk

    a. Avoiding discontinuation of suicide watch without a proper risk assessment

    b. Giving proper consideration of warning by family

    c. Gathering information from correctional staff before the clinician meets with the inmate

    d. Timely communication by mental health professional with the correctional staff after suicide risk assessment

4. Suicide watch monitoring

    a. Performing accurate suicide watch on a staggered basis

    b. Accurate documentation of suicide watch log

5. Classification and housing of inmates

    a. Placing at-risk inmates in suicide-resistant cells which contain no materials for self-harm

    b. Receiving input from mental health staff for housing inmates

    c. Minimizing isolation and avoiding solitary confinement when possible

6. Adequacy of psychiatric treatment

    a. Avoiding delay in treatment

    b. Avoiding abrupt discontinuation of medication

    c. Providing bridge medication

    d. Adherence to substance-withdrawal protocols

7. Monitoring inmates in administrative segregation and special housing
8. Development and implementation of suicide prevention policy
    a. Periodic review of the policy implementation and practice
    b. Making sure abnormal practice and procedures do not become well settled to the detriment of inmates
9. Establish adequate mental health services delivery system
    a. Timely access to mental health services
    b. Prompt response to MSR
10. Adequate staffing of correctional staff and mental health staff
11. Consistent and adequate training of correctional and mental health staff
    a. Training and documentation of suicide prevention training for all new staff
    b. Training and documentation of routine annual suicide prevention training for all staff

CONCLUSION

Systematic and rigorous adherence to policy, procedures, and practice by correctional administrators, custody staff, and clinicians promotes the safety and security of suicidal inmates and mitigates third-party claims. Consistent, systematic, and scheduled repeat training of the staff is critical.

REFERENCES

1. Ross, D. *Liability Trends in Suicide in Jails, Prisons and Lockups,* American Jails (2010)
2. Farmer v. Brennan, 511 U.S. 825 (1994)
3. Miranda v. County of Lake, 900 F.3d 335 (7th Cir. 2018)
4. Comstock v. McCrary, 273 F.3d 693, 6th Cir. (2001)
5. Williams v. Mehra, 186 F.3d 685 (6th Cir. 1999)
6. Greason v. Kemp, 891 F.2d 829 (11th Cir. 1990)
7. Steele v. Shah, 87 F.3d 1266 (11th Cir. 1996)
8. Estate of Ryan Clark v. County of Green Lake, No. 14-C-1402, 2016 WL 4769365 (E.D. Wis. Sept. 13, 2016)
9. Gordon v. Kidd, 971 F.2d 1087 (4th Cir. 1992)
10. Freedman v. City of Allentown, 853 F.2d 1111 (3d Cir. 1988)
11. Conn v. City of Reno, 658 F.3d 897 (9th Cir. 2011)
12. Simmons v. Navajo County, 609 F.3d 1011 (9th Cir. 2010)
13. Minix v. Canarecci, 597 F.3d 824 (7th Cir. 2010)
14. Broughton v. Premier Health Care Services, Inc., No. 15-4150 (6th Cir. July 15, 2016)
15. Strickler v. McCord, 306 F. Supp. 2d 818 (N.D. Ind. 2004)
16. Terry v. Rice, CAUSE No. IP00-0600-C K/H (S.D. Ind. Apr. 18, 2003)
17. McKee v. Turner, No. 96-3446, 1997 WL 525680, (6th Cir. August 25, 1997)
18. Jackson v. West, 787 F.3d 1345 (11th Cir. 2015)
19. Cavalieri v. Shepard, 321 F.3d 616 (7th Cir. 2003)
20. Estate of Novack v. County of Wood, 226 F.3d 525 (7th Cir. 2000)
21. Steele v. Han Chul Choi, 82 F.3d 175 (7th Cir. 1996)
22. Gutierrez v. Peters, 111 F.3d 1364, 1371 (7th Cir. 1997)

23. Hunt v. Dental Dept, 865 F.2d 198 (9th Cir. 1989)

24. Harris v. Coweta County, 21 F.3d 388 (11th Cir. 1994)

25. Goodloe v. Sood, 947 F.3d 1026 (7th Cir. 2020)

26. Gomez v. Randle, 680 F.3d 859, 865 (7th Cir. 2012)

27. Perez v. Fenoglio, 792 F.3d 768, 777–78 (7th Cir. 2015)

28. Forbes v. Edgar, 112 F.3d 262, 267 (7th Cir. 1997)

29. Quinn v. Lashbrook, No. 18-cv-2013- RJD (S.D. Ill. July 9, 2020)

30. Mitchell v. Kallas, 895 F.3d 492 (7th Cir. 2018)

31. Greeno v. Daley, 414 F.3d 645, 654–55 (7th Cir. 2005)

32. Durmer v. O'Carroll, 991 F.2d 64, 69 (3d Cir. 1993)

33. Wambold v. Varner, CIVIL ACTION No. 3:14-2206, at *2 (M.D. Pa. January 15, 2019)

34. Arenas v. Ga. Dep't of Corr., No. CV416-320 (S.D. Ga. Feb. 20, 2018)

35. Norfleet v. Webster, 439 F.3d 392 (7th Cir. 2006)

36. Estate of Cole v. Fromm, 94 F.3d 254 (7th Cir. 1996)

37. Palakovic v. Wetzel, 854 F.3d 209 (3d Cir. 2017)

38. Braggs v. Dunn, 367 F. Supp. 3d 1340, 1344 (M.D. Ala. 2019)

39. Frey v. City of Herculaneum, 44 F.3d 667, 670 (8th Cir. 1995)

40. White v. Watson, No. 16-cv-560-JPG-DGW (S.D. Ill. October 26, 2016)

41. Bd. of the Cty. Commissioners of Bryan Cty., Okla. v. Brown, 520 U.S. 397, 410 (1997)

42. Gibson v. County of Washoe, 290 F.3d 1175, 1189 (9th Cir. 2002)

43. Gates v. Cook, 376 F.3d 323, 333 (5th Cir. 2004)

44. City of Canton, Ohio v. Harris, 489 U.S. 378 (1989)

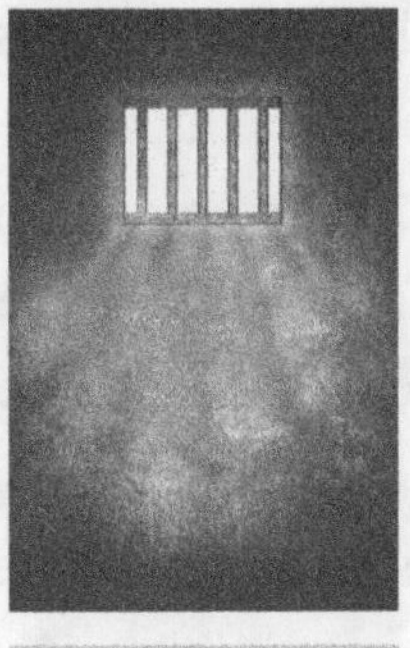

CHAPTER 8

EXPERTS IN SUICIDE-RELATED LAWSUITS

In our adversarial system of justice, experts play a critical role to assist the trier of fact (jury or judge) in reaching legal decisions. The experts in correctional practice generally represent a wide variety of domains, including medical and mental health care, jail and custody practice, administrative organization, and policies, procedures, and practice. The commonly retained experts include correctional physicians and psychiatrists, forensic psychiatrists and psychologists, nurses and nurse administrators, jail and police experts, wardens, administrators, and sometimes academicians and suicide researchers.

Experts, by their experience, skill, training, education, and expertise, impart specialized knowledge to the judge and the jury on health and mental health practices, jail and prison policies and practices, the standard of care, deliberate indifference,

227

and on any matters relevant to the lawsuits involving suicide, wrongful death, and serious injuries.

An expert witness is a person retained by attorneys representing plaintiffs or defendants to offer opinions by reports, deposition, and/or declaration in anticipation of litigation or during trial. In many cases, the expert works as a consultant before he/she becomes an expert witness.

Expert analysis, study, opinions, and testimony are governed by the Federal Rules of Evidence 702* and its components. The rules state that expert opinions are admissible if the expert's scientific, technical, or other specialized knowledge will help the trier of fact to understand the evidence or to determine a fact at issue. The testimony must be based on sufficient fact or data, analyzed by valid and reliable methodology.

STANDARDS OF EXPERT OPINIONS

Expert opinions must meet the following standards:

1. Reliability
2. Relevance to the issue in the lawsuit
3. Helpfulness to the jury and/or the judge

The side that offers the expert carries the legal burden for laying the proper foundation for the admission of the expert opinions and testimony in court. The offeror, plaintiff, or defendant must ensure that the expert meets the qualification requirements to testify competently, that he or she relies on sound methodology, and that the proposed testimony will help the trier of fact to understand something that is beyond the knowledge of the average juror. [1, 2]

Reliability

Reliability of opinions depends on the use of valid and generally accepted methods designed to analyze the data related to each case scenario. The expert must apply the methods reliably to the facts of the case. The method used must ensure the results are dependable and accurate. The trial court examines and reviews the methodology the expert uses in reaching conclusions. In other words, the trial court functions as a "gatekeeper to ensure speculative and unreliable opinions" are kept out of jury deliberations.[1] Challenging expert opinions by questioning the methodology the expert used and its reliability is commonly known as a Daubert challenge on the recognition that any opinion based on an unreliable method must be unreliable as well.

The expert must be able to explain the methodology and principles supporting the opinions. He/she must describe the nature and type of data considered and how they are analyzed, how the results are reached, and how the opinions are formed. In other words, opinions must be more than mere conclusions. If these essential criteria are not met, the expert's opinion should be ruled inadmissible by the court. In *Wendler v. AIG, Inc.*,[3] the court found an expert's report inadmissible because the expert failed to specify what method was used, the data considered and results produced, and how alternative explanations were ruled out.

Relevance

The trial court determines whether the expert opinions are directly relevant to the issue raised in the legal complaint of a lawsuit. If the litigated issue is medical negligence, the opinions must be relevant to the issue (i.e., whether the health care professional, by acts of commission or omission, deviated from the standard of care). The expert may opine on the services provided or not provided, and all issues related to the standard of care. The opinions may include the status of the officials' credentials, qualifications, and training.

In certain cases, the court may allow the expert to opine on standard of care in special settings such as administrative segregation in correctional setting. In *White v. Watson*[4] the court opined, "the experts qualified to opine on the standard of care governing a correctional officer's treatment of an inmate in segregation may testify as to the standard of care." The court further opined that "they may be examined and cross-examined about hypothetical sets of facts, but they may not express an opinion on which alternate set of facts is true or on the credibility of any witness to support either set of facts," or express opinions on other matters a jury is clearly qualified to determine itself. It is axiomatic that experts are not permitted to opine on the credibility of witnesses.

In *Terry v. Rice*[5] the court held that the experts must have the necessary qualifications and should be familiar with standards of care in correctional and medical practice. They must be able to articulate their opinions regarding negligence and what constitutes deliberate indifference. The court noted that the experts did not attempt to define explicitly the legal term "deliberate indifference" but they discussed the facts of the case and concluded that the facts amounted to deliberate indifference. They did not conclude whether the prison officials were deliberately indifferent to the inmate's serious medical need. The court emphasized that a finding and conclusion if the deliberate indifference occurred is a fact question for the jury.

Helpfulness

Expert opinions must be helpful to the trier of fact. The courts routinely disallow speculative opinions because they are not helpful to the jury in arriving at a just decision. Therefore, expert opinions inferred from speculation about the mental state of a correctional official involved in a deliberate indifference lawsuit should not reach a jury.[6]

Another significant issue disallowed by the court involves the testimony on the conclusions of the law. Directly opining that a defendant acted with deliberate indifference is tantamount to making a legal conclusion that addresses the ultimate question of the lawsuit because it usurps the province of the jury.[5]

Federal Rules of Evidence 704 Advisory Committee Notes show that "testimony offering nothing more than a legal conclusion—i.e., testimony that does little more than tell the jury what result to reach—is properly excludable under the Rules." It is also appropriate to exclude "ultimate issue" testimony on the ground that it would not be helpful to the trier of fact when "the terms used by the witness have a separate, distinct, and specialized meaning in the law different from that present in the vernacular."

Rules 704, 701, and 702 of the Federal Rules of Evidence provide ample protection against inadmissible opinions. Rule 704(a) states: "testimony in the form of an opinion or inference otherwise admissible is not objectionable because it embraces an ultimate issue to be decided by the trier of fact." For example, the expert may opine that a health-care provider deviated from the standard of care or what actions, or inactions constituted the deviations, but should not opine that the provider was medically negligent. Rules 701 and 702 state that opinions must be helpful to the trier of fact. These provisions afford ample assurances against the admission of opinions which would "merely tell the jury what result to reach."

The Woods court[6] held that an expert could not testify that the defendant acted with deliberate indifference because that mental state was an element of the alleged statutory violation. Furthermore, the court opined, any testimony which tells the trier of fact the results expected or what conclusions to be reached is not only not helpful but also inadmissible.

Stacking an inference on another inference and then stating an opinion regarding the ultimate issue is less likely to be helpful to the trier of fact. Opinions must be supported by facts, which form the basis of opinions. If not, the court will reject testimony, either during a deposition or during trial.

In *Burkey v. Hunter*,[7] plaintiff's expert Murray's report and deposition testimony were found unreliable and unhelpful to the jury. The decedent in the case was on the top floor of a parking garage with one foot on the ledge two days before he committed suicide in the Mahoning County Jail. Before he was admitted to the jail, he was seen at St. Elizabeth Hospital's ER, where a nurse determined he was suicidal based on suicide screening. As a result, he was placed on suicide precaution in the emergency room. He was released to Mahoning County Jail with the recommendation that he be placed on suicide watch. However, the information that he was suicidal and required suicide precautions was never conveyed to the jail personnel.

Expert Murray opined in his report and deposition testimony that the "administrators and staff at Mahoning County Jail were aware of the risk of suicide and there was an expectation for a viable jail suicide prevention program." He opined about system failures including "the many ways by which the actions of Jail personnel failed to meet basic expectations" of a suicide prevention program. He then concluded that "the staff failures coupled with the noted systemic problems takes this situation beyond negligence to a level of deliberate indifference." He stacked speculation upon speculation and opined that the County engaged in deliberate indifference to the inmate suicide. Murray, however, failed to opine how an individual officer knew or should have known that the decedent had a strong likelihood of suicide and how individual officers failed to take any action to mitigate the decedent's risk.

While not challenging that the decedent had a sufficiently serious medical need, Officers Hunter, Vath, and Peters contended that none of them knew any facts from which they could infer that the decedent was a substantial suicide risk.

Therefore, the court opined that without evidence of defendants' subjective knowledge of decedent as a substantial suicide risk, Murray's opinion that Mahoning County staff acted with deliberate indifference was unsupported by the evidence in the record. Accordingly, the court did not consider Murray's expert witness report and deposition testimony reliable and helpful to the jury.

In *Cook Ex Rel. Tessier v. Sheriff of Monroe County*[8] the plaintiff did not establish that expert Dr. Maris's testimony would assist the jury, and, therefore, that his testimony was inadmissible. He listed ten opinions but did not elaborate the basis of his opinions. The opinions included:

1. Monroe County failed to accurately assess Tessier's suicidality despite his two to three written requests for psychiatric treatment. Also, Monroe County's mental health and suicide assessment forms were inadequate to detect Tessier's mental illness, alcohol abuse, and prior suicide ideation.
2. Because the County policy showed that jail suicide occurs within 72 hours, Tessier should have been placed on close observation.
3. One-hour checks were "grossly insufficient" to prevent jail hangings, and Monroe County's suicide prevention training procedures were unclear and inadequate to prevent jail suicides.
4. Had Tessier seen a psychiatrist and been treated for anxiety and depression he would not have committed suicide.
5. An officer should have read Tessier's request for treatment.
6. The jail had an excessive number of suicides.
7. The jail failed to correct, modify, or otherwise change serious suicidogenic conditions at the jail.
8. The cells were not suicide proofed.
9. Monroe County was "deliberately indifferent to Tessier's serious medical needs and violated Tessier's constitutional right to not suffer cruel and unusual punishment, by ignoring his written requests for psychiatric treatment and evaluation."

10. If Monroe County had "responded appropriately and promptly to Tessier's psychiatric condition, it is more likely than not that he would not have committed suicide."

Maris's opinions reveal several flaws. He did not identify whether Tessier was at suicide risk at any time, whether the jail officials failed to recognize Tessier's risk when it was present, and whether they failed to take action to mitigate his risk. The expert opined the forms were not sufficient to capture Tessier's history of mental illness and substance abuse but failed to link the deficient form to Tessier. And even though suicides in a jail mostly occur within 72 hours of arrival, that does not mean that an inmate can be placed under close suicide observation unless he makes suicidal statements, has risk factors that place him at heightened risk for suicide, or the officers perceive or determine him to be at suicide risk. It was pure speculation for the expert to opine that Tessier would not have committed suicide if he had been seen in response to his requests. He opined about the policies and training without linking how the perceived lack of training to any officer or a mental health professional affected Tessier. Finally, he directly opined that the County was deliberately indifferent and violated Tessier's constitutional right, which is, of course, a legal conclusion.

ADMISSIBILITY OF RECORDS

Inmate records are official records of business and, therefore, they are likely to be admissible in court. They are not hearsay evidence if they meet the requirements stipulated by Federal Rule 803(6). In *Wheeler v. Sims*[9] and *Terry v. Rice*,[5] the courts indicated that a prison or jail is considered a business for the purposes of Rule 803.[6] Any records created in the normal course of conducting the business are considered as business records. The records must fulfill certain requirements to be considered as business records:

1. The person with knowledge of the prison or jail creates the record.
2. The creation of the record is the regular practice of the prison or jail as a regularly conducted business.
3. The records are the types of official business records authorities keep in the usual course of running a jail or prison.
4. The entries are recorded at or near the time of their occurrence.
5. A custodian of record authenticates the records for them to be considered as certified.

EXPERT ANALYSIS

Experts in suicide-related litigation face unique challenges that include lack of a standard method, technique, or formula in performing analysis and study.

The analysis of a claim depends on whether the litigation is about medical negligence and/or deliberate indifference. For a negligence claim, the analysis focuses on whether a health-care provider deviated from the standard of care and such deviation had any nexus to the injury or death of the inmate.

In contrast, analysis of a deliberate indifference claim is a more complicated process. This may involve a review of the administrative structure, staff organization, contracts with the providers, policies, procedures, and practices concerning access to medical and mental health care, and suicide prevention, as well as monitoring of care and staff training and any other aspect of care. The goal is to determine whether the correctional organization and the staff, having known the serious medical and mental health needs of an inmate, deliberately disregarded such needs, which caused or contributed to his injury or death.

Method of Analysis

1. *Records*

An expert generally agrees to consult on a case after he or she determines a lack of conflict of interest with the parties involved. The complexity of the lawsuit and, sometimes, lack of organization of the related documents, dictates the amount of time and effort required to analyze and study the case.

The retaining attorney obtains the documents through a process known as discovery after a lawsuit is officially filed. If an attorney fails to provide documents the expert needs, it is the duty of the expert to request such documents to complete the study.

Often, the documents include the inmate's (the subject in the case) jail or prison records, medical and mental health records, policies and procedures, mental health and medical manuals, and depositions of the sued parties and officials, and custody providers and administrators. In addition to the legal complaint filed in the court, the documents for review will include judicial records such as interrogatories and answers to interrogators by both sides and other related discovery materials.

The records commonly relied upon to complete an objective case analysis include:

1. Medical and mental health records of the subject (inmate)
    a. Jail/prison intake and booking form
    b. Reports from arresting officer
    c. Jail/prison health screening form
    d. Suicide screening form
    e. Mental health evaluation and progress notes
    f. Physician orders
    g. Medication Administration Records
    h. Suicide watch logs
    i. Administrative segregation reviews and logs
    j. Past psychiatric records and requests for those records
    k. Communication from family members
2. Correctional records
    a. Classification file
    b. Grievance forms and resolution
    c. Inmate movement log
    d. Medical Services Request forms
    e. Record of action taken following Medical Requests
    f. Control room logs
    g. Video recordings of the jail and hallways
    h. Photographs of the cell where suicide attempt occurred
    i. Crime scene photographs and videos
    j. Any other written communications including emails that include reference to the inmate

3. Coroner's report
   a. Postmortem report of the decedent
   b. Toxicology report of the decedent
4. EMT reports (if any)
5. Post-suicide attempt hospitalization records
6. Investigative reports
   a. Internal investigation
   b. Root cause analysis
   c. Psychological autopsy
   d. External investigation
   e. Morbidity and Mortality review, if available
7. Facility mental health manual
8. Facility policies and procedures
   a. Suicide prevention
   b. Access to mental health care
   c. Psychotropic medication
   d. Medication administration
   e. Classification and housing
   f. Administrative segregation
9. Contractors' records
   a. Contract between the vendor and the facility
   b. Contractors' policies and procedures
10. Training-related documents
    a. Training curriculum (course of study) and sylla-bus (subjects covered)
    b. Training logs
11. Legal documents
    a. Complaint and subsequent amended iterations, if any
    b. Interrogatories and response to interrogatories

12. Depositions of various parties involved including:
    a. Officers
    b. Health and mental health providers
    c. Administrative representatives
    d. Designated individuals knowledgeable about policies and procedures
    e. Trustees and other inmates
13. Personnel files of involved providers
    a. Curriculum vitae
    b. License and certifications
    c. Disciplinary file
14. Other documents
    a. Citizens review board report (if any)
    b. Department of Justice monitor reports
    c. Special Master's reports as applicable
    d. Special Master's depositions

2. *Review Process*

A correctional expert retained to consult on a suicide-related litigation may choose to rely primarily on the documents pertaining to his/her specific professional area of expertise. However, the expert must get an overview of the case before rendering opinions.

- A jail/prison policy expert may concentrate on officers' entries and practice, video evidence and policies.

- A psychiatrist may lay particular emphasis on risk identification, risk assessment, psychiatric practice, and related policies.

- A correctional nurse expert may choose to determine whether the nurses involved in the case complied with nursing standards, medication administration, and related practice.

- An administrative expert may selectively review the overall structure and organization, contracts, mental health service delivery, and policy and procedure development and implementation.

- A forensic psychiatric expert with correctional and administrative experience may rely on entire documents and evidence.

Experts must perform an objective review and examination of health-care and suicide screening documents, correctional records, mental health and medical records, applicable policies and procedures, administrative directives, state statutes and codes, and testimonies to determine whether the facility health-care professionals and correctional officials complied with standards of practice and procedures or committed acts of omission and commission that can be interpreted as deviation of the standard of care and/or a conscious, reckless disregard of the inmate's suicide vulnerability.

The expert analyzes not only the specific aspects of care provided to the inmate but also the facility's overall structure and organization to determine whether reasonable care was provided to inmates to support or refute a claim.

Then, the expert applies his/her hands-on experience, specialized knowledge, and research in arriving at a logical and reasoned set of observations, findings, and professional opinions. Since the subject of the lawsuit is deceased, no direct examination is feasible.

a. *Assembling facts*

The expert gathers case details of the inmate (the decedent and/or the serious suicide attempter) from the records. The details include demographics, date of occurrence of the critical incident, method of suicide attempt or suicide, post-incident correctional staff, and medical intervention and hospitalization, if any. Some jail and police policy experts visit the facility to inspect the cell where the critical incident occurred.

At the outset of the review, the expert focuses on identification of the risk factors the inmate presented before the critical event. The documents that provide the information on risk factors include screening questionnaires, suicide risk assessment, mental health and psychiatric evaluation, chronology of care, arresting officers' report(s), correctional officer's observations and entries, suicide watch logs, family member's reports, past jail records, past psychiatric outpatient and hospitalization records, the inmate's statements, correctional officials' entries and incident reports, and physician and nursing entries.

Retrospective identification of substantial risk factors that caused or contributed to a strong likelihood that the inmate would have attempted suicide is a major challenge. By reviewing the records, including the deposition testimonies of involved officials, the expert attempts to establish whether the inmate had specific and substantial risk factors. They include, but are not limited to, a history of recent near-lethal suicide attempt/s, or a progressive trajectory of suicidal behaviors, active suicidal ideation with intent and plan during detention, active mental illness with psychotropic medication use, substance withdrawal, a history of suicide among the first-degree relatives, a mental state of hopelessness and a narrowing of interests, anxiety, agitation, and psychosocial stressor acting as a precipitant of suicide.

b. *Subjective awareness of inmate's risk*

The expert then determines the officials' (mental health professionals and correctional officers) subjective awareness of the specific risk factors and of the inmate's particular suicide vulnerability. The expert bases such a determination on objective evidence in the records of the inmate's substantial suicide risk factors, behavior, and suicide statements, plan, and intent.

The fact that a suicide occurred or was attempted does not necessarily mean that the officials deviated from the standard of care or failed to act to mitigate the inmate's risk of harm. It could be that the officials did not know that an inmate was at risk.

c. *Deviation from the standard of care and deliberate indifference*

Upon finding that the official knew or should have known the inmate's suicide vulnerability, the next step involves determination of what the official did or did not do to mitigate the inmate's risk. Here, the expert concentrates on specific action that the official was reasonably expected to take to mitigate the risk. Based on the available evidence, the expert determines if the official deviated from the standard of care and/or if the standard is deliberate indifference, disregarded the inmate's risk by failing to provide appropriate intervention, monitoring, and treatment.

The expert makes specific determination of the following domains:

1. Did the jail/prison official apply the best practices in identification and assessment of the inmate's suicide vulnerability?

2. Did the jail/prison official apply the best practices in intervention, monitoring, and treatment of the inmate?

3. Did the jail/prison official, having known the inmate's suicide risk, disregard it by not taking any steps to mitigate the risk?

4. Did the jail/prison official act consistently with the facility's policies and procedures?

5. Did the jail/prison official fail to follow the policies and procedures and did such failure contribute to or cause the inmate's suicide attempt?

d. *Monell claims analysis*

The principal step involved in Monell claim review is analysis and study of the jail/prison policies, procedure, or practice and programs. As the court in *White v. Watson*[4] indicated, the policies, procedures, or the custom must be the "moving force" in the failure to protect an inmate. The expert specifically attempts to determine any causative link between policies and programs, particularly the manner and method of implementation and practice and inmate injury or death.

The causation analysis pertaining to Monell claims requires a review of the following documents:

1. The facility's programs and policies on:
   a. inmate access to mental health services
   b. psychiatric treatment; and
   c. compliance with suicide prevention measures
2. Suicide watch monitoring and logs
3. Crisis monitoring

4. Administrative segregation logs
5. Staffing pattern
6. Staff training and supervision
   a. Suicide training syllabus and curriculum
   b. Training schedule
   c. Officials' training attendance logs
   d. Officials' license and credentials
7. Private vendor contract compliance
8. Federal monitoring reports

   e. ***Proximate relationship***

Upon determination that the official deviated from the standard of care or disregarded the inmate's suicide vulnerability, the final step in the process of expert review and study involves formulation of opinions to establish a causative link, (i.e., proximate relationship between the failures and critical incident).

The expert must establish specifically how an individual jail/prison official deviated from the standard of care and/or violated the inmate's constitutional rights. Courts have particularly indicated that a claim of constitutional violation must be made against an individual official (Chapter 7) although courts have considered global inadequacy of care in determining validity of Monell claims.

On the other hand, the record may show evidence of how an official acted reasonably to address an inmate's suicide vulnerability. The expert must pay attention to the evidence and the possibility that it compels the conclusion that the official did not have any knowledge of the inmate's suicide risk.

WRITING PROFESSIONAL OPINIONS

The most important tool to express the expert's opinions is a professional report of the study and analysis. Upon completing the study, the expert must prepare a well-reasoned and thorough report outlining all opinions. The expert renders his or her opinions with a reasonable degree of professional certainty or probability (i.e., more likely than not). The opposing counsel will scrutinize the report for any holes or flaws so that they can use them to discredit the expert.

The United States District Trial Court's procedures are governed by Federal Rules of Civil Procedure (FRCP). FRCP Rule 26 mandates that an expert witness produces a written report of his/her opinions that meet specific standards. In some jurisdictions the expert may be banned from testifying if the report does not meet the Rule 26 stipulations. Some courts may have additional requirements. These may be available in local rules that may be obtained online or from the court clerk. The purpose of the report is to avoid any surprise opinions during trial. The expert must make the report available to the retaining attorney who will serve the report on opposing counsel and, in some jurisdictions, file it with the court clerk before a deadline set by the court. For a state court case, the report requirement varies from state to state. For such cases, the expert should verify the requirements with the retaining attorney.

DISCLOSURE OF EXPERT TESTIMONY

Rule 26(a)(2) states:

(A) In General. In addition to the disclosures required by Rule 26(a)(1), a party must disclose to the other parties the identity of any witness it may use at trial to present evidence under Federal Rule of Evidence 702, 703, or 705.

(B) Witnesses must provide a written Report. Unless otherwise stipulated or ordered by the court, this disclosure must be accompanied by a written report—prepared and signed by the witness if the witness is one retained or specially employed to provide expert testimony in the case or one whose duties as the party's employee regularly involve giving expert testimony. The report must contain:

(i) a complete statement of all opinions the witness will express and the basis and reasons for them;

(ii) the facts or data considered by the witness in forming them;

(iii) any exhibits that will be used to summarize or support them;

(iv) the witness's qualifications, including a list of all publications authored in the previous 10 years;

(v) a list of all other cases in which, during the previous 4 years, the witness testified as an expert at trial or by deposition; and

(vi) a statement of the compensation to be paid for the study and testimony in the case.

FORMATTING AND COMPOSING THE REPORT

A well-prepared report is highly organized in style and content. The report must be done professionally on personal or business letterhead with no typographic errors or grammatical mistakes. It must be composed in single page copy and properly paginated. If necessary, have someone with proofreading skills review the report before finalizing it. The expert must affix a handwritten signature and date the report.

Experts must write in active prose in such a manner that it is easily understood by a layperson and must explain technical jargon to the extent possible. He or she must avoid speculation, exaggeration, hyperbole, and puffed-up opinions.

Proper heading and subheadings will facilitate easy assimilation of facts, figures, and statements. Avoid all hedge words and phrases such as "it appears"; "apparently"; "somewhat"; "it seems"; "essentially"; and the like. Each paragraph, succinctly prepared, should contain one idea or one opinion and supporting statements.[10]

In composing the report, the expert may include a few paragraphs at the beginning of the report, outlining his or her specific qualifications relevant to the case at hand, though he or she should attach a complete curriculum vitae to the report.

The report must contain a complete statement of all opinions in the case and the basis of the opinions. The report must address the specific issues the retaining attorney has asked, and any issues raised in the legal complaint. All conclusions and opinions must be supported by facts and data considered by the expert. If any data does not support his opinions, he should give an explanation as to why it was rejected. The expert may furnish a supplemental report if additional facts or documents become available, depending upon the judicial time schedule of the case.

A current curriculum vitae accurately summarizing the expert's accomplishments, positions, qualifications, publications, awards, presentations/speeches, licenses, and other relevant professional details must accompany the report. Usually, publications for the past ten years included in the curriculum vitae will be sufficient instead of providing a separate bibliography.

If reference to specific citations is made in the text of the report, it will be appropriate to append a bibliography specific to the report. If any article or scientific materials are referenced in the expert report, they must be based on valid studies, peer reviewed, and published in reputable journals. Opinion pieces and editorials have less usefulness as supporting references.

The report in a federal case must list all cases in which the report's author testified during the previous four years. Every expert must keep track of all cases in which he or she testified by deposition or in trial. The list must provide sufficient details of the cases including the title and case number, location/venue, name of the presiding judge, date testified, and, if possible, central issues of the case. The expert is not required to list the cases in which he or she consulted but did not testify.

Finally, the expert must include his or her fee schedule, compensation received for the study and testimony, and estimates of the fee for future work.

Components of a high-quality expert report related to suicide case analysis and study may vary depending on the type of the case. However, besides the Rule 26 requirements, it must contain the following:

1. A complete listing of all documents considered. Specifically, the documents listed must be identified by date, source, and if possible, by Bates number.

2. Details of the case, including the demographics of the decedent (or the severely injured), a summary of the critical incident, and the events surrounding the suicide attempt and post-attempt lifesaving measures
3. Identification and description of the main issues or questions raised by the retaining attorney and those listed in the complaint
4. Suicide and health-care screening data
5. Description of the events preceding the inmate suicide, details of care, and correctional officers' observations
6. Suicide watch, logs, and monitoring records
7. Findings from the investigative report
8. Video matrix outlining the significance of what is shown on the video
9. Consistency of officers' actions with policies, procedures, and regulations in place at the time
10. Training schedule, curriculum, and personnel data

This section generally should not include any opinions, though some analytical data may be included.

OPINION SECTION

A plaintiff expert report should reflect valid, data-supported opinions consistent with parameters of deviation of the standard of care and/or deliberate indifference. The expert may prefer to use the term "conscious disregard" of serious medical need in place of deliberate indifference.

Many experts confuse deviation from the standard of care (i.e., medical negligence) with constitutional violation. This misconception arises from the fact that inmates have a constitutional right to adequate (reasonable) medical and mental health care. Therefore, some experts may incorrectly opine that any deviation from the standard of care involving inmate mental health and medical care may be the same as violation of constitutional rights.

When addressing deviation from the standard of care involving an at-risk inmate, experts must opine how a provider deviated: what he did or did not do that caused or contributed to the injury or death of an inmate. Many deviations from the standard of care regarding diagnosis, assessment, monitoring, and treatment do not carry an element of intentionality or willfulness. On the other hand, in some cases gross omission or commission of acts may show conscious disregard of the medical and mental health needs of an inmate sufficient to support the deliberate indifference standard for constitutional claims.

The constitutional right to medical and mental health care does not entitle an inmate to a specific treatment or what is desirable. Therefore, expert opinions indicative of differences in medical judgment or type of treatment chosen if such substituted medical decisions do not have the potential to harm the inmate may not support either a medical negligence or a deliberate indifference claim.

Statutory and code violations are not the same as deviations of the standard of care nor, standing alone, are they grounds for a deliberate indifference claim. State statutes and administrative codes establish the requirement of policies concerning correctional practices including a suicide prevention program, and qualifications of mental health professionals and their role. However, they do not set the standards of medical/psychiatric care and suicide risk identification and assessment.

Expert opinions on deliberate indifference must address the involved correctional official's subjective awareness of the inmate's strong likelihood of suicide, based on substantial risk factors and whether the official disregarded such a risk and all issues related to it. He or she must identify how a correctional official knowingly withheld action/s or ignored responsibility that existed for him or her in their professional capacity. Opinions supporting deliberate indifference must include evidence that the official knowingly withheld a professional action or did not take a required action. It does not require proof of intent to do harm to the inmate. However, the expert opinions must indicate an official's appreciation of the potential for a substantial negative outcome.

If the lawsuit involves a medical professional, the opinion may include how he or she did or did not exercise reasonable and appropriate professional judgment to mitigate suicide risk.

Suppose an expert opines that global failure to sustain an adequate mental health service delivery system in a facility impacted inmates. Collective failure means that every staff member in a system or facility failed, but to opine that everybody was responsible for a failed mental health system devalues an expert's opinion because such a scenario seldom exists. Human error or accident is not evidence of deliberate indifference.

The opinions may also involve all aspects of the correctional officials' (correctional officers and mental health professionals) training, qualification, and credentials.

If the lawsuit involves a Monell claim, the expert may opine on the type and nature of training and supervision of the officials, and how training and supervision impacted the at-risk inmates. If the training program departed from the acceptable industry standard, then the opinions may focus on how *objectively unreasonable* those practices were and how such practices impacted screening, identification, and assessment of inmates at potential risk. Likewise, opinions may center on how a de facto custom or practice was "*the moving force*" or driving force that caused or contributed to the risk of an inmate.

Based on the case law analysis noted in Chapter 7, expert opinions may center on one or more of these scenarios: inadequacy of mental health evaluation by a provider; failure to identify obvious and substantial risk factors; officers' failure to communicate an arrestee's suicide statements; failure of suicide watch procedures; failure to consider a prisoner's recent suicide attempt; and failure to get prior medical records. Opinions may include diagnosis and treatment issues such as inadequate treatment, inadequate diagnosis, intentional refusal of treatment, delay or inadequate treatment, and policy, staffing, and training.

Opinions may cover solitary confinement and monitoring, continued placement in segregation, medication non-compliance, and vulnerability factors such as sudden mental status changes including anxiety, agitation, insomnia, and hopelessness. Scheduling delays, failure to complete suicide risk assessment and screening forms and incident reports, failure to place an inmate on suicide risk, lack of policy compliance, and failure to recognize suicide risk given an inmate's history of suicide attempts may become the subject of an expert's opinions. Failure to adhere to "watch take" medication dispensation, allowing an inmate to hoard medications, and not maintaining a suicide watch cell bereft of anchor points should receive an expert's attention. Other areas include an officer's undue delay in taking an inmate down from hanging, letting an inmate hang while the camera is located, and failure to transfer an inmate to a crisis stabilization unit and/or to inpatient unit. Opinions may cover staffing patterns and training schedule and curriculum. Finally, warning by family members of a loved one's risk, if documented, must receive the expert's attention.

Like the plaintiff's experts, the defense's experts must provide valid and data-supported opinions. Opinions may center on the strengths of mental health services delivery, adequacy of suicide prevention policy, procedures and practice, and conduciveness of facility's organization and staffing patterns to suicide prevention. Opinions may highlight the staff training and curriculum. More specifically, defense expert may opine how the psychiatric services and risk identification and assessment were adequate and appropriate and that any claim of deviation of standard of care and deliberate indifference have no bearing to the injury and death of the inmate. A defense expert may argue that the correctional official did not know the inmate's suicide risk (if that is the case). Sometimes, a defense expert would have access to the plaintiff's expert's report and, if so, directly, or indirectly respond to his/her opinions.

Occasionally, a rebuttal report to address any disagreement with the opposing expert may be required. Rule 26 (a)(2)(D) permits a report "solely to contradict or rebut evidence on the same subject matter" within 30 days after the opposing party's expert disclosure. The opposing expert's opinions can be contradicted, not necessarily to establish that the expert opinions are wrong, but to indicate a different viewpoint. Sometimes, a rebuttal report may be used to rehabilitate the retained expert's opinions while discrediting the opposing expert's opinions. The rebuttal report should not contain new opinions or contradict the expert's original report.

CONCLUSION

In summary, the experts in suicide litigation must adhere to the highest standard of analysis and study, follow reliable methodology, and write an objective report outlining his or her opinions consistent with Rule 26's requirements.

REFERENCES

1. Daubert v. Merrell Dow Pharm., Inc., 509 U.S. 579, 599 (1993)
2. Allison v. McGhan Med. Corp., 184 F.3d 1300, 1306 (11th Cir. 1999)
3. Wendler Ezra, P.C. v. Am. Int'l Group, Inc., 521 F.3d 790, 791 (7th Cir. 2008)
4. White v. Watson, 2018 WL 4326998 No. 16-cv-560-JPG-DGW, at *6–7 (S.D Ill, 2018)
5. Terry v. Rice, CAUSE No. IP00-0600-C K/H (S.D. Ind. Apr. 18, 2003)
6. Woods v. Lecureux, 110 F.3d 1215, 1220 (6th Cir. 1997)
7. Burkey v. Hunter, No. 4:17CV338 (N.D. Ohio Feb. 27, 2019)
8. Cook Ex Rel. Tessier v. Sheriff Monroe Cnty, 402 F.3d 1092, 1109 (11th Cir. 2005)
9. Wheeler v. Sims, 951 F.2d 796, 802 (7th Cir. 1992)

10. Joseph, J. *Composing Expert's Report: Factors for Compliance with Federal Rules 26(a)(2)(B)*. Journal of Handwriting.com 31 (2013)

* The Federal Rules of Evidence are a set of rules that govern the introduction of evidence at civil and criminal trials in United States federal trial courts.

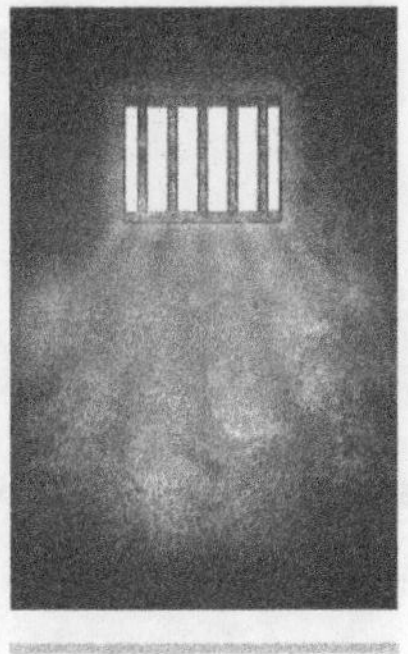

CHAPTER 9

LIFE AND COURSE OF A SUICIDE-RELATED LAWSUIT

A *Cornell University Law School study* shows that 94,496 civil lawsuits were filed on behalf of prisoners in the U.S. between 2012 and 2018.[1] The study does not identify the type of lawsuits, (i.e., prisoner or next of kin-initiated malpractice, deliberate indifference, prisoner class action lawsuits, or other causes). Sixty-seven percent were settled out of court, and 33% went to trial. However, according to a Department of Justice report published in 2004,[2] 97% of all civil cases filed in state and federal courts were settled or dismissed without a trial. According to the report, the number tried in court fell from 22,451 in 1992 to 11,908 in 2001. Plaintiffs won 55% of the cases and received $4.4 billion in damages. Government statistics, recent or past, specifically related to suicide in jails and prisons were not available. (The high non-trial-based resolution

259

is consistent with my personal experience of lawsuits in jails and prisons.)

U.S. COURT SYSTEM

The United States court system is an overlapping network of different courts. They are divided into federal and state courts, and each system is divided into several layers.

Most state courts comprise probate, family, and circuit courts, with an upper tier of appellate courts and the state supreme court. State courts handle both civil and criminal cases. The probate division deals with wills. Family courts handle divorce, custody, and related matters.

The next tier of the court system is the appellate court, which addresses whether the lower court made any serious errors of law.

The federal court system has three levels: district courts, circuit courts, and the U.S. Supreme Court. There are ninety-four district courts, thirteen circuit courts, and the Supreme Court.

A plaintiff has the initial option to bring a case in state court or a federal court. Federal district courts are the trial courts in the federal system. They handle both criminal and civil cases. Some tasks in a district court are assigned to magistrate judges, who are appointed for a term of eight years, instead of district court judges, who are lifetime appointees by the president. Magistrate judges sometimes handle summary judgment and Daubert motions involving suicide-related lawsuits.

The circuit courts hear appeals from the district courts from their respective regions. Each federal court of appeals issues decisions that have precedential power over the courts within its circuit. Once there is a federal jurisdiction, the federal court will also hear supplemental state law claims that go with a case asserting deliberate indifference with medical malpractice appended to it.

Circuit judges are presidential lifetime appointees. Appeals to circuit courts are filed as briefs, arguing why the trial court judgment should be affirmed or reversed. Then, a panel of three circuit judges hears oral arguments from attorneys representing both sides before rendering its judgment.

The Supreme Court of the United States is the highest court in the land. A case decided by the federal circuit court, or any state Supreme Court can appeal to the U.S. Supreme Court. A party may file a "writ of certiorari" asking the Supreme Court to hear the case. However, unlike the circuit court of appeals, the Supreme Court is not required to hear the appeals. The most common basis for the Supreme Court's accepting a case is to resolve a split among the circuit courts. If the writ is granted, briefs will be filed like those of the circuit court of appeals, then the Supreme Court will hear oral arguments before rendering its decision. If the writ is not granted, the decision by the lower court stands. The Supreme Court comprises nine justices and takes judicial precedence over all other courts in the nation. A judgment by the U.S. Supreme Court applies to the entire country.

Below I note the routes taken by state and federal cases to get to the Supreme Court:

State trial court >> State Appellate Courts >> State Supreme Court >> U.S. Supreme Court

Federal District Courts >> U.S. Court of Appeals >> U.S. Supreme Court

JUDICIAL EVENTS

In a civil lawsuit, the plaintiffs' lawyer begins a lawsuit by filing a complaint at the district court. Today, most complaints are e-filed via the ECF (Electronic Court Filing) system. If the court permits, the initial complaint can be amended a few times before the trial.

Once the court accepts the filing, the next step is service upon the named defendants, followed by the defendants filing their answer/s to the complaint or a motion to dismiss. At this point, the issues are considered "joined." If the defendants fail to respond, a default judgment is issued for the plaintiff.

The next phase of the lawsuit is the discovery phase. Both parties engage in written discovery seeking potential evidence that includes interrogatories, requests for admissions, and requests for production of documents.

The court sets a judicial calendar of pretrial events, including a discovery deadline, a date by which the parties must submit dispositive motions, and a deadline for submitting expert reports. The court may also set a date for mediation and settlement efforts. The court initially sets the date of the final pretrial motions, jury selection, and the trial.

After they submit their reports, retained experts are usually deposed, but they will testify in court only if the case goes to trial. It is interesting to note that retained experts appear at trial in only about 10% of their cases throughout the country.

In the federal court, an expert report must include a complete statement of all opinions the witness will express and the basis and reasons for them; the facts or data considered by the witness in forming them; any exhibits that will be used to summarize or support them; the witness's qualifications, including a list of all publications authored in the previous ten years; a list of all other cases in which, during the last four years, the witness testified as an expert at trial or by deposition; and a statement of the compensation to be paid for the study and testimony in the case. (See Chapter 8)

In a jury trial, weeks before the jury is seated, a pretrial conference will take up issues immediately relevant to the trial. Typically, during the pretrial conference, which involves the judge and the respective attorneys, the court will take up motions *in limine*, Daubert motions, and pretrial objections to proposed witnesses, exhibits, jury instructions, and *voir dire* questions. The court also requires the parties to meet to confer and attempt to resolve motions involving discovery disputes.

A party may file a motion in limine to limit or exclude certain evidence or arguments to be presented by the opposing counsel during trial. In Latin, *limine* means "the threshold," and the threshold is the beginning of the trial. Specifically, the motion is intended to prevent the introduction of irrelevant, inadmissible, or prejudicial matters. The judge handles the motion outside the presence of the jury. Federal rules of evidence govern the motions in limine. Rulings on motions in limine do not exclude evidence but prohibit either party from offering the disputed testimony during trial prior to obtaining an evidentiary ruling.

Pretrial disclosures include witness list, deposition designations, exhibit list, proposed jury instructions, and *voir dire* questions.

The party using video depositions during the trial is responsible for preparing the final edited video in accordance with their party's designations and the court's rulings on objections.

The party that proposes to offer deposition testimony shall serve a disclosure identifying the line and page numbers to be offered and must file the deposition with the court by a designated date.

Expert witness designation and report due date

The court sets the due date for expert witness reports. First, the party with the burden of proof will produce its experts' reports. Experts designated by the opposing side must then produce their reports on a designated date that is set by the court or agreed to by the parties. Supplemental reports may be permitted if new information arises after the preparation of the original report.

Some district courts permit parties to designate a rebuttal expert witness/s who may produce rebuttal reports; most do not. If a party serves a supplemental expert report without prior agreement after the rebuttal expert report deadline has passed, the serving party must file a notice with the court. The filing must state that service has occurred and why a supplemental report is necessary under the circumstances and the reason for seeking leave to supplement the report.

Jury Trial

In a jury trial, the phases of the trial comprise (1) *voir dire* (2) opening statements (3) direct and cross-examinations, and (4) closing arguments. In French, *voir dire* means "to see to speak." It is a process by which attorneys can reject a juror to be seated on the jury panel. In a state court, both sides ask questions of the potential juror to determine whether they are competent and suitable to serve on the jury panel. In federal court, the parties submit proposed questions to the judge, but only the judge questions the jurors. Each side may suggest that certain potential jurors be dismissed "for cause," meaning some close involvement with a party or with a previous similar situation that makes it unlikely that the juror can render an unbiased verdict. After dismissals for cause, each side may exercise a designated number of preemptory strikes for which no reason need be given. The jurors who remain comprise the jury.

After the jury is seated, the trial begins with opening statements by attorneys representing both sides, followed by examining witnesses via direct and cross-examination. After the presentation of evidence, closing arguments by the parties are completed. The case then goes to the jury.

In some districts, the trial is bifurcated, meaning that first, the jury will determine only whether one or more defendants has violated a plaintiff's rights. This is the liability phase. If the jury returns a verdict in favor of all defendants, the trial is over. If the jury returns a verdict finding any or all defendants liable, the trial continues in order to reach an agreement on the issue of damages. After damages evidence, the jury again retires to determine what amount the plaintiff should receive for their injuries and whether to assess punitive damages against any defendant.

Expert Deposition

An expert deposition is an out-of-court record of the expert's opinions, taken under oath. It carries the same weight as the testimony during a trial, except that a judge is not physically present during the deposition but technically available to make a ruling on a disputed issue.

There are two types of deposition: evidentiary deposition and discovery deposition. Evidentiary deposition serves the purpose of preserving evidence for trial. The questioning during evidentiary deposition is limited, while the scope of discovery depositions is quite broad.[3] As with discovery, generally, the subject of depositions can range from any nonprivileged matter that is relevant to any party's claim or defense. The scope of the deposition is determined solely by relevance under Rule 26, that is, that the evidence sought may lead to the discovery of admissible evidence.[4] Rule 26(b) provides that "[p]arties may obtain discovery regarding any matter, not privileged, that is relevant to the claim or defense of any party . . . Relevant information need not be admissible at the trial if the discovery appears reasonably calculated to lead to the discovery of admissible evidence."[5]

The opposing attorney takes a discovery deposition of an expert with multiple goals:

1. To know the expert's complete opinions
2. To size up the expert as a witness
3. To gather ammunition to discredit or impeach the expert during trial
4. To file pretrial motions such as motion in limine, or a Daubert motion
5. To use the contents of the deposition to secure a summary judgment

EXPERT AT DEPOSITION

Besides maintaining professional etiquette and appropriate attire, the expert must listen carefully to the questions by the attorney and take adequate time to respond to them. The expert must allow the attorney to complete his or her questions. It is natural to anticipate the next question and answer before the attorney completes a question. This will not only interfere with any objection that the retaining attorney would raise, but also the intended question might be different from the one anticipated.

The expert must not argue or engage in a shouting match with the attorney. Instead, he or she must remain calm and collected and answer questions in a dignified manner.

Preparation is the key in providing well-reasoned opinions in full. The expert must know the case thoroughly, express his/her opinions confidently, and defend all of those opinions. When answering questions, the expert must avoid absolute terms such as "never" or "always" as well as hedge words such as "I guess" "it appears" and "I estimate" or similar words, but allow enough wiggle room to respond to questions on new documents or information.

Sometimes an attorney may twist the expert's words, misstate facts and other witness statements, or distort or confuse policies with standards. If the deposing attorney assumes that the expert agrees with the premise of a question, he/she may seek answers that he/she likes, but not necessarily the one the expert intends to provide. Active listening is the best strategy to respond to such questions.

Rule 26 requires experts to furnish their curriculum vitae, fee schedule, and cases testified during the previous four years. As such, the line of questioning would cover the expert's qualifications, credentials, employment history (particularly gaps in employment), faculty appointments, courses taught, disciplinary actions, and terminations. Unfortunately, some attorneys may try to shock the experts at the outset of the deposition by highlighting any negative personal and professional information to throw the expert off his/her composure.

The expert will be asked about the nature of their professional practice, particularly the percentage of time in clinical or correctional practice, administrative role, and research. More specifically, the expert will be asked the percentage of time devoted to expert work and its earnings. This line of questioning may establish any break in the expert's employment or career or if the expert is continuously engaged in his/her customary line of work. For example, if the expert exclusively engages in expert witness practice, an attempt to portray the expert as a "professional" witness will be made.

Questions often cover the expert's license, board certification, disciplinary action against the license, lawsuits against him/her, and the outcome. In addition, if the expert is an international medical graduate, the deposing attorney may question the standing of the expert's college, university, naturalization, and citizenship status.

Credibility is the only thing that the expert has. Jeopardizing credibility is detrimental to the expert's career. Therefore, the expert must opine truthfully, fully, and to the best of his/her ability, consistent with the oath taken at the beginning of the deposition.

The expert should not opine on the credibility of a witness, but rather, the testimony should be about the reliability of data in the documents to formulate his/her opinions.

Almost every expert has a website. While the questions center on the expert's advertisement of his/her expertise and services, more important, the website content will be used to establish any outlandish claims and inconsistencies in the expert opinions.

Billing and time spent on reviewing the documents and report writing will be the focus of the attorney's inquiry. In addition, the expert may be asked the estimated fee for additional work, including future testimony during the trial.

The expert will be asked about previous engagements by the retaining attorney and his/her firm. Also, the expert will be questioned about number of times he or she has testified previously in suicide-related lawsuits and the percentage testified for plaintiffs and defense.

Inquiry on opinion formation

The deposing attorney may inquire when the retaining attorney contacted the expert, what was exchanged during the initial contact, and if the attorney asked for a specific opinion on the case. Ordinary practice involving an attorney's first contact with an expert comprises the attorney introducing the case, a general discussion of the expert's expertise on custodial suicide and correctional practices, including mental health and medical care, and a discussion of the expert's interest in consulting on the case. It will be appropriate for the expert to reject a case if an attorney seeks a specific opinion or directs him/her to provide opinions before the expert conducts their analysis and study. Attorneys seeking an expert will use their own criteria to select an expert. (See appendix 4)

Timing of opinion formation will be a line of inquiry. In the normal course of analysis and study, as the expert reviews the documents, it is only natural for the expert to form preliminary impressions, not necessarily opinions that require confirmation or rejection. The expert must consider every relevant fact by reviewing all documents forwarded to him or her. If a critical document is missing, the expert should seek such a document from the retaining attorney. The expert will be questioned whether he/she has sought to obtain any relevant missing documents and if they were received.

Another line of inquiry involves whether the expert reviewed any documents after completing the report. Sometimes, the expert may receive the opposing expert's report and deposition and any other deposition of parties taken after submitting the report. The questions will then involve whether the expert modified his/her opinions or formed new opinions in considering the additional documents. If new opinions were formed, a supplemental report, within the constraints of the judicial calendar (if the court permits) should be issued.

The expert will be questioned on whether he or she consulted any literature and whether such literature is authoritative on the subject matter of the case. The expert's publications will be likely quoted to determine the consistency of opinions with the contents of those publications. As the information in any article or literature evolves over time, it will be appropriate to opine that the literature provides valuable information, but the expert may stop short of declaring it as authoritative. Suppose the expert has identified any specific literature or article or the expert's own research and publications. In that case, questions may involve the methodology and whether the data and conclusions were peer-reviewed and generally accepted by other experts in the field.

The deposing attorney may use published materials by national organizations such as the American Psychiatric

Association (APA), the American Correctional Association (ACA), and the National Commission on Correctional Health Care (NCCHC) to examine the expert. The expert must be familiar with such publications. If presented at deposition, carefully read them before answering questions about information included in such documents. The expert must determine whether they are mandates, guidelines, or suggestions. The organizational standards are usually guidelines that leave an opening for the expert to evaluate them before answering the questions carefully. NCCHC standards may support generally accepted practice. For instance, standard J.E.07 shows that the inmates should have the opportunity to submit daily Medical Service Requests (MSR) and those slips are to be picked up and triaged. NCCHC standards are not mandatory. They are recommendations, but compliance is expected.

Sometimes, the expert may be questioned if he or she has talked to the plaintiff/s or the defendant/s. Ordinarily, experts do not talk with any involved parties, including the injured inmate who filed the lawsuit.

If an expert visited the jail where the suicide or serious suicide attempt occurred, information regarding such a visit might become a focus of inquiry.

A line of inquiry may include the materials/documents that an expert brought along at deposition. Nowadays, most documents are available digitally. However, some experts may bring all documents on a specifically assigned device such as a laptop or iPad.

An attorney may meticulously question the expert on the methodology of the analysis and study. Any excluded key data may be the focus of inquiry to see if such data was intentionally excluded. The inquiry may center on the records reviewed, who provided them, and when.

Expert's notes of review of the records can be a focus of questioning about when the notes were made, and at what point in relation to the notes the expert formed an opinion or opinions.

Questions on preparation for deposition may include documents reviewed, when and how long, meetings with the retaining attorney, new documents reviewed, and any new opinions formed. While the contents of the conversation between the expert and the attorney may be considered as a work product, it may be appropriate to acknowledge such conversations and duration.

A focus would be whether the expert's prior testimony was ever limited or excluded, or the expert was disqualified, and any successful Daubert motions.

A tactic would be to use previous depositions to establish any inconsistency in the testimony in the current case, though the previous case was different from the present one. If the expert cannot recall his/her previous testimony, it is advisable to ask the attorney for the transcript of the prior testimony, then carefully review it before answering questions. Because each case is different, the expert may emphasize what distinguishes the present case from the previous testimony—without being "evasive, defensive, or untruthful."[6] Unless the current case is identical to the prior case, which is unlikely, the best way to handle such questioning would be to make a statement such as "I agree generally, but the current case" is different for certain reasons.

As the deposing attorney questions the expert, a line of inquiry would be on what is included in the report and what is not, trying to establish that the expert may have intentionally or unintentionally left out some key data. In addition, the deposing attorney usually asks about each stated opinion and the supporting explanations. The attorney may question the expert's opinions at the outset of the deposition, or may follow the outline of the expert's report.

Finally, the deposing attorney will try to establish that the expert used unreliable methodology or methods that are not generally accepted in the field and that the expert did not rely on any standards, statutes, and codes, laying the foundation for motions to limit or exclude the expert's testimony later.

OPINION INQUIRY

I share my experience and lessons learned by providing at least nineteen depositions on suicide-related lawsuits and the topics attorneys cover during depositions. I have also reviewed at least one hundred depositions by other correctional experts.

The deposing attorney may spend considerable time questioning the expert about his/her opinions because of the critical role expert opinions play in the outcome of a lawsuit. Most attorneys who specialize in suicide-related litigation are well prepared and knowledgeable in the legal, and, to a significant extent, the clinical issues involved in these lawsuits. The experts will be best served if they have a working knowledge of the legal aspects of the case, including negligence, medical negligence, deliberate indifference, ADA issues, and state statutes and administrative codes pertaining to policy development and mental health employees' qualifications.

Experts must be prepared to agree to generally accepted theories, positions, and generalizations related to correctional and mental health practice. They must concede or admit those issues that are obvious and consistent with the correctional standard of care. Generally accepted standard-of-care issues include reviewing the inmate's prior records, particularly of those who attempted suicide in the past, in determining an inmate's suicide risk. Not taking an inmate's denial of suicidal ideation at face value is another area where experts agree. The practice of asking an inmate directly about suicidal ideation, plan, and intent is standard practice.

Likewise, placing an inmate on suicide precautions upon identifying potential risk of harm, having a mental health professional perform suicide risk assessment, and having a qualified mental health professional discontinue suicide precautions are universally accepted practices. An officer placing an inmate on suicide watch if the inmate makes a suicide statement or his/her behavior suggests suicide risk is the standard.

Phenomenological aspects of inmate suicide often become the focus of inquiry. They include the definition of suicide ideation, plan and intent, suicide attempt, suicidal behaviors and manipulative attempts, and distinction among terms such as actively suicidal, imminently suicidal, and acutely suicidal (inmate) and the transient nature of suicidal ideation. In addition, questions may cover the percentage of inmates with suicidal ideation who take their lives compared with past suicide attempters. Finally, questions may include if suicide can be predicted and whether risk factors have any predictive value.

The attorney may depose the expert if he or she has formulated an opinion regarding screening questionnaire-based determination of the inmate's suicide risk and placement on suicide watch. Questions may center on the scope and comprehensiveness of the suicide screening questionnaire, risk determination, communication by the screener with the mental health staff, documentation of assessed risk, and the data collection procedure. Because there is compartmentalization between correctional and mental health staff in a facility, failure of communication between the two regarding inmate risk determination could be the basis of intense examination of the expert.

Method of suicide risk assessment, type, and comprehensiveness of the data gathered to complete a reasonable and medically supported risk assessment, time spent by the mental health professional performing the risk assessment, and qualifications and training of the professional are salient areas of inquiry. Suppose a contractor of mental health services employs an unlicensed mental health professional to perform suicide risk assessment. In that case, the training type, scope, and supervision level will form the basis of additional questions.

Specifically, the attorney will inquire how the supervision of the professional was provided and his/her competency assessed. In addition, the attorney will attempt to establish that the professional's training was inadequate and, therefore, any assessment performed by inadequately trained person was inadequate as well.

Assessment of the degree of suicide risk would be a major issue in determining the level of precautions, type of monitoring, and choice of treatment inmates require. Therefore, the attorney may vigorously question the level of risk determined by the correctional officers and the official's steps to mitigate such risk. More important, the attorney may give special attention to the mental health professional's decision to discontinue suicide precaution, as well as the manner, circumstances, and mechanics of assessment that resulted in the discontinuation of precautions. In addition, questions to determine if the professional gathered reasonable information from the correctional officers and reviewed the jail or any mental health records and whether the professional appropriately communicated his/her decision to the shift commander follow.

Another area of inquiry would be about communication by family members to jail/prison personnel of potential risk to the inmate. Questions will cover when the correctional officials received those messages, what actions resulted from such messages, and if those messages had any impact on decision-making.

Sometimes, the duration of contact by a mental health professional with the inmate performing a suicide risk assessment may become the focus of intense examination. While there is no standard duration for a suicide risk assessment, the deposing attorney will highlight the extremely limited face-to-face contact with the inmate. Here, the deposing attorney would attempt to establish that the suicide risk assessment was inadequate because the mental health professional did not take time to consider all the risk and protective factors. The implication, therefore, would be that any decision to discontinue the precaution was flawed, which directly contributed to the death of the inmate.

While a plaintiff's deposing attorney would try to establish that the defendant's mental health professional performed an inadequate suicide risk assessment, the defendant's deposing attorney would point out the assessment's strengths.

Statistics of suicide and suicide attempts have often become the focus of inquiry, particularly about facilities with a history of multiple attempts and suicides. Experts must be prepared to respond to questions on the suicide rate in jails and prisons in general, and specifically in the facility where the lawsuit was based.

The attorney will ask about the structure, quality, and the type of mental health services delivery and its relation to suicide in the facility. In addition, questions may cover the implementation of policies and procedures if the suicide rate exceeded the average in the facility, regionally or nationally, during several years before the (plaintiff's) death and, more specifically, in the year the inmate died. The purpose of this line of inquiry is to establish that the facility administration knew of any critical deficiencies and failed to remedy those that could be directly linked to the correctional officials' awareness of the decedent's risk.

Speaking of the mental health services delivery, the expert should be familiar with the structure, organization, and staffing required to deliver adequate mental health services in the facility. More importantly, inadequate staffing has a direct relationship to inmate suicide. Questions on whether correctional setting would make any difference in suicide risk assessment and treatment modalities are common. Limitations and budgetary constraints inherent in correctional practice may allow the experts to opine that a certain type of treatment, for instance, typical psychotherapy, is not commonplace in a correctional setting.

Experts must be prepared to opine on specific inmate behaviors and statements and their proximity to (plaintiff) suicide. In addition, the experts will be queried on what a correctional official knew about the inmate's suicide vulnerability and if they knew it in relation to the suicide. Questions on what specific actions the official took or failed to take to mitigate such risk will follow. If the official failed to take any action, the expert will be asked what specific action a prison official should have taken. For instance, questions may include placing an inmate on suicide watch, prescribing, arranging for medications, transferring to a crisis stabilization or an inpatient unit, or any other mitigating steps. Questions would also cover if the correctional official had a subjective awareness of the inmate's potential risk and, if so, what actions he or she took—or failed to take—to mitigate the risk.

The totality of circumstances of a decedent, adequacy of care or lack thereof, and system deficiencies can be significant issues.

Suppose the inmate (decedent) had certain psychiatric disorders that increase their lifetime risk of suicide. In this instance, opinions showing that because the (decedent) had psychiatric disorder/s, the inmate should have been placed on suicide watch or admitted to a psychiatric inpatient unit, lack specificity. The (plaintiff) inmate must express suicidal thoughts or demonstrate behaviors indicative of suicide risk or have mental states including depressed mood, anxiety, hopelessness, and agitation immediately preceding the suicide. While a non-suicidal mentally ill inmate should be provided adequate psychiatric treatment with medications or referral to a psychiatric unit, failure to take such steps alone is not consistent with reckless disregard of the serious medical need of that inmate. At issue should be the identification of suicide risk and failure to take action to mitigate that risk.

The impact of substance withdrawal and associated symptoms and their relation to suicide may become the focus of inquiry. The expert will be questioned if the provider considered the inmate's substance abuse and withdrawal effects in suicide risk assessment and if so, what actions the provider took or failed to take to deal with the inmate's substance abuse and withdrawal. Additionally, the attorney may explore alcohol, opiate, and benzodiazepine withdrawal, and their relationship with suicide.

Experts must be able to testify on the scope, content, and adequacy of facility policies. In addition, the attorney will question whether any practice and custom had become well established to the extent that they became the driving force to deprive the inmate of his/her constitutional rights.

The training curriculum, schedule, and staff attendance in the training program will often become the subject matter in a case. The purpose of this line of questioning is to establish that the training of the facility officials was inadequate and therefore, the care provided to the inmate in question was inadequate, linking the inadequate training to the suicide.

Delay in medical and psychiatric care is particularly relevant in some lawsuits. Experts must be able to opine on triaging of MSR, appointment scheduling practice, and how any delay has contributed to the inmate's suicide. In addition, experts must be able to opine on the NCCHC standard related to access to mental health care and related matters.

Psychiatric experts should be familiar with medications, prescription practice, physician orders, Medication Administration Records, pharmacokinetics, dose and administration routes, and medication side effects if medication treatment issues are a concern in a case. The correctional health-care-specific practice of "bridge" medications, "watch take," and "keep on the person" practice may be relevant in some cases. If a correctional officer dispenses medications in a facility, their training and supervision will be a focus of inquiry.

A correctional nurse expert must be familiar with nursing standards, MAR, transcription of physician orders, medication dispensation and documentation, side effects, and MSR.

It is inadvisable to testify on standards of a profession not belonging to him/her—for instance, nursing standards if the expert is a non-nurse. However, the expert may appropriately testify about correctional procedures and practice, including the practice of suicide watch procedures, an officer's decision to place an inmate on suicide watch, and inmate safety checks and logs. Likewise, the expert may testify on the practice of medication dispensation and communication issues between nursing and correctional officers.

Deposition questions may include placement of inmates in administrative segregation and mental health monitoring and documentation. Other subject areas of intense questioning may include special-needs inmates, indications and practice of crisis watches, and classification and inmate housing assignment procedures.

In some instances, deposition inquiry may involve internal investigations such as psychological autopsy, "root cause analysis," and the expert's opinions on them.

DAUBERT STANDARD AND CHALLENGE

The Daubert standard comes from the Supreme Court case, Daubert v. Merrell Dow Pharmaceuticals Inc.[7] Under the standard, the factors that may be considered in determining whether the methodology of analysis and study is valid are:

1. Whether the theory or technique in question can be and has been tested
2. Whether it has been subjected to peer review and publication
3. Its known or potential error rate
4. The existence and maintenance of standards controlling its operation
5. Whether it has attracted widespread acceptance within a relevant scientific community

In *General Electric v. Joiner*[8] the Supreme Court clarified *Daubert*, holding that an appellate court may still review a trial court's decision to admit or exclude expert testimony. The standard of review for this inquiry is the abuse of discretion standard (if the discretionary decision by the lower court was made in plain error).

In *Kumho v. Carmichael*[9] the Supreme Court further clarified that the Daubert factors may apply to non-scientific testimony, meaning "the testimony of engineers and other experts who are not scientists."

Any party may move to strike expert opinions, asserting that the expert is not qualified, or that the opinions are not relevant or reliable, or that opinions invade the province of the jury by purporting to render conclusions of the law. Once such a challenge is made, the expert has the burden to prove by a preponderance of the evidence that the opinions expressed in the report and testimony are both relevant and reliable.

Common challenges include implications that the expert's opinions are not based on facts. For example, making a sweeping statement on the suicide risk of an inmate without reliably identifying risk factors and without linking officials' lack of inference of the inmate's suicide risk, and not specifically identifying how the prison officials ignored such a risk can be the basis of a challenge. Experts must avoid speculations at any cost. Experts also must be careful not to engage in making credibility determinations of witnesses.

Opinions expressed in the report must be consistent with the opinions expressed during deposition. Defendants will highlight any inconsistencies between the report and deposition testimony to discredit the opinions. In addition, most courts will not permit an expert to testify to any opinion that was not part of his/her report.

Opinions on system failures and substandard care without specific and direct involvement by the officials in the decedent's care may be another challenge.

Parties may dispute the expert's opinions expressing conclusions of law that invade the province of the jury and the court. Specifically, a conclusory opinion that prison/jail officials were deliberately indifferent to an inmate's serious medical need will lead to a challenge. Therefore, the expert may preferably describe the prison officials' failure to take specific actions that could be interpreted as reckless or conscious disregard without specifically opining that they committed acts of deliberate indifference.

Another issue that can be raised would be providing opinions without reference to any standards, regulations, practice, or code within the field of corrections. Certain techniques and methods are so common and accepted that they may not be rooted specifically in identifiable standards but have become part of common vernacular in the correctional practice. For instance, questioning an inmate on suicidal ideation is generally accepted as a standard practice. It is understood that the safety and security issues in a facility become an overriding concern, with the result that individual concern for privacy becomes a secondary issue. However, the expert should be able to articulate standards as outlined by the NCCHC and the officials' failure to comply with national standards. The expert's experience and expertise acquired by working in jails and prisons is another avenue to face these challenges if such experience is limited in scope.

The defendant may raise an issue to question the expert's methodology to determine emotional pain and suffering. Some jurisdictions require opinions on pain and suffering that the decedent experienced before his death to permit the jury to consider awarding compensation. There is no uniformly accepted methodology available to the expert with which he could have reached his conclusion that an inmate suffered from undue emotional stress and pain at the time of his hanging, immediately preceding his death, or for days to weeks before his death. However, physicians by training, education, and experience ought to have knowledge and expertise to assess emotional stress and pain at the time of or before inmate hanging.

Properly performing the expert analysis based on technical, scientific, and specialized knowledge of the subject matter—suicide vulnerability, a serious medical need, and applying the acceptable methodology to analyze the data and facts to render opinions to assist the trier of fact—will help to avoid any Daubert challenge.

SUMMARY JUDGMENT

Expert testimony is crucial to avoiding (or winning) summary judgment (a judgment entered by a court for one party and against another party without a full trial) in matters requiring expert testimony. That sounds syllogistic, and probably is, but it's also important. Few cases ever go to trial, often because a defendant wins a summary judgment. Solid expert testimony is crucial in both cases. Summary judgment may not be granted if the evidence shows there's a genuine issue (conflict) of material fact concerning the claims. Since the expert witness plays something of a dual (fact/legal) role, expert opinion is often treated as "fact." If there's a conflict, summary judgment will be denied.

Summary judgment is appropriate where the court is satisfied "that there is no genuine issue as to any material fact and that the moving party is entitled to a judgment as a matter of law."[10] A fact is material only if it affects the outcome of the case. A dispute of material fact is "genuine" if the evidence is such that a "reasonable jury could return a verdict for the non-moving party."[10] The court grants summary judgment "if the pleadings, depositions, answers to interrogatories, and admissions on file together with the affidavits (if any), show that there is no genuine issue as to the material fact that the moving party is entitled to a judgment as a matter of law."[11]

The burden of establishing the nonexistence of a "genuine issue" is on the party moving for summary judgment. The moving party's burden has two distinct components: first, an initial burden of production to establish a prima facie case by producing sufficient evidence that there is no genuine issue and second, an ultimate burden of persuasion. The court must not decide whether the moving party has satisfied its ultimate burden of persuasion unless and until the court finds that it has discharged its initial burden of production.[12]

In *Lewis v. Cnty of Northumberland*[13] expert opinions played a significant role in the court's decision on a summary judgment motion filed by the defendants that included the County of Northumberland and a private vendor of mental health services at the jail.

Cyrus Lewis was arrested after a motor vehicle accident, driving under a suspended license. He was taken to a local hospital, but he left the hospital unauthorized. He was arrested the next day. He told the officers that he wanted to end his life.

The suicide screening questionnaire indicated that the arresting officer believed that he was suicidal. As per the questionnaire, he was at high risk of suicide. He was placed on suicide watch Level I in a cell with anchor points, and given his clothes and sheets.

A social worker employed by the private health care agency contracted with the jail performed a behavior health assessment the day after his detention. She noted he did not have a good support system and he had a history of bipolar depression and past hospitalizations. She further noted that he was not accepting of his incarceration and was argumentative with her. He was not sure about his future but contracted for safety, agreeing not to do anything harmful to himself. He told her that he was an IV drug user and an alcoholic with a history of rehabilitation. On the second day of detention, after he verbally denied suicidal ideation, she changed his level of suicide watch from a higher Level I to lower Level II.

The social worker saw him again the next day. He was still withdrawing from alcohol and heroin. He denied suicidal ideation and stated there was nothing wrong with him psychologically. He contracted for safety. She decided to continue him on Level II.

The social worker saw him the day after. She noted that his mood was less dysphoric, his affect was less flat, he was "future-oriented," and he had good eye contact. As a result, she decided to change the level of supervision from II to III.

A day later, Lewis expressed a suicide wish to a defendant correctional officer and to two inmates. An inmate told the defendant officer that Lewis was talking about killing himself. The officer asked the inmates to watch him.

The same day, the defendant officer found Lewis hanging with a sheet tied to a windowsill at the back wall in his cell.

During the preceding six years Lewis had a significant psychiatric history, including multiple psychiatric hospitalizations for suicidal ideation, attempts, depression, and substance abuse.

The jail had three levels of suicide watch in addition to constant observation, which is reserved for actively suicidal inmates. The jail's suicide prevention policy stated that the staff "shall observe such a patient on a continuous, uninterrupted basis and have a clear, unobstructed view of the patient always. Observation shall be documented at 10-minute intervals."

Level I Suicide Watch: This level was reserved for those not actively suicidal but who expressed suicidal ideation and had a plan to commit suicide. They were considered at medium to high risk of suicide. They were issued a suicide-resistant smock and suicide-resistant blanket. At this level, the staff "shall observe the patient at random, staggered intervals, not to exceed 15 minutes" by direct visual observation. This level was also used for inmates at high risk.

Level II Suicide Watch: This was a step-down from Level I. Patients on this level were issued a jumpsuit or jail uniform, shoes without shoelaces, a mattress, and a suicide-resistant blanket. They were placed in a stripped cell with no underwear, socks, sheets, sharps, and belts and were observed at intervals not to exceed 15 minutes on a staggered basis.

Level III: This was considered psychiatric observation. It was not used for suicide prevention; it was reserved for patients whose behavior warranted close observation. They were observed at intervals not to exceed 30 minutes on a staggered basis. They had all the rights and privileges of an inmate in the general population.

Based on analysis and study of all documents, I opined that, despite his denial of suicidal ideation with the social worker, Lewis was of high suicide risk throughout his detention, presenting with substantial and obvious risk. He was placed in a cell with anchor points and materials with which he could hang himself. I further opined that he was not given a psychiatric evaluation to establish proper diagnoses and treatment plan. Such an evaluation was warranted and medically necessary because of his history of depression, specifically major depressive disorder, anxiety disorder, substance dependence, and use of antidepressant and antianxiety medications.

Health-care standards applicable to correctional health-care settings demand that a proper psychiatric evaluation is conducted within a reasonable period when inmates enter a jail or prison. Such a reasonable period is within 14 days of admission. However, it is expected that such evaluation is completed within 72 hours when an inmate has a known history of mental illness, medication use, and high suicide risk. In his case, the social worker failed to schedule a psychiatric evaluation.

The social worker took Mr. Lewis's denial of suicide ideation at face value when she changed his level of supervision from Level II (watch every 15 minutes) to Level III (watch every 30 minutes) on the day of his suicide. I opined that the change from Level II to Level III was not only premature but was a deviation from the standard of care of patients/inmates with significant suicide risk. The social worker was fully aware of his risk, disregarded his risk, and changed his level. Placement of the decedent in a cell with anchor points with bedsheets and clothing, knowing well that he was of substantial and obvious suicide risk, indicated a lack of professional judgment to his serious medical need.

The defendant officer knew that Lewis expressed a wish to kill himself. She did not communicate his status change, (i.e., imminent suicide risk), to mental health providers.

The special security check was suspect because of its regularity at every 15 minutes. The defendant officer, in fact, did not perform the security check and falsified the logs. Such dereliction of duty is a reckless disregard of the inmate's expressed serious suicide risk.

After the defendants received the expert opinions, the County and the private vendor of mental health services filed a motion for summary judgment.

The court considered expert opinions of both defendant and plaintiff experts. In the summary judgment order, the court opined that "medical expert testimony is properly considered for the purpose of summary judgment in the context of deliberate indifference claims," citing *Estate of Kempf v. Wash. Cnty.*[14]

In denying the summary judgment motion, the court took into consideration the expert report of "Dr. A.E. Daniel who determined that the (decedent) posed a significant suicide risk at the time he was booked and remained so throughout the confinement at (prison); the placement of the (decedent) in a cell with known anchor points with bedsheets and clothing, knowing his obvious and substantial risk, amounted to deliberate indifference; that the defendant (officer) knew that he was expressing suicidal ideations, did not communicate his status change, and instead asked two inmates to watch him; that defendant (officer's) security check was suspect because of its regularity and because of the testimony of two inmates and at least one officer regarding the (officer's) conduct at work. Dr. Daniel further opined that (social worker's) "change of the decedent's status from Level II to III was not only premature but also a clear deviation from the standard of care of patients/inmates with significant suicide risk, but that (social worker), despite being fully aware of this risk changed his level anyway."

The court noted that suicide vulnerability of the decedent was based on five factors: opiate withdrawal, most recent suicide attempt (the vehicle crash was considered a suicide attempt), the decedent's classification as a high risk, his placement on suicide watch, and his expression of suicidal intent. Suicide must be a strong likelihood, rather than a "mere possibility that the inmate may commit suicide."

The court further opined that "viewing material facts in the record in a light most favorable to plaintiff the court finds that a reasonable jury may find that both sets of defendants knew or should have known Lewis's particular vulnerability to suicide and were deliberately indifferent to that vulnerability."

Lewis's case was settled after the summary judgment.

CONCLUSION

Although they face challenges, experts play a crucial role in the life and course of a suicide-related lawsuit. Ultimately, their role is to analyze the data, provide objective opinions, and assist the officers of the court and the trier of fact to determine the outcome of the case.

REFERENCES

1. https://scholarship.law.cornell.edu/cgi/viewcontent.cgi?article=1202&context=facpub
2. https://www.bizjournals.com/phoenix/stories/2004/05/31/newscolumn5.html)
3. Hickman v. Taylor, 329 U.S. 495, 507–508 (1947)
4. Overseas Private Investment Corp. v. Mandelbaum, 185 F.R.D. 67 (D.D.C. 1999)
5. Paasewe v. Anjana Samadder, M.D., Inc., No. 2:04-cv-724 (S.D. Ohio (February 27, 2006)
6. Babitsky, S and Mangraviti, J: https://www.testifyingtraining.com/how-to-excel-at-your-expert-witness-deposition/ SEAK, Inc, (2015)

7. Daubert v. Merrell Dow Pharmaceuticals Inc. 509 U.S. 579 (1993)

8. General Electric v. Joiner, 522 U.S. 136 (1997)

9. Kumho Tire Co. v. Carmichael 526 U.S. 137 (1999)

10. Anderson v. Liberty Lobby, Inc., 477 U.S. 242 (1986)

11. Farrell v. Planters Lifesavers Co., 22 F. Supp. 2d 372 (D.N.J. 1998)

12. Celotex Corp. v. Catrett, 477 U.S. 317 (1986)

13. Lewis v. Cnty. of Northumberland, CIVIL ACTION No. 4:14-CV-02126, at *2 (MD Pa. December 15, 2016)

14. Estate of Kempf v. Wash. Cnty, 2:15-cv-00486-TFM (W.D. Pa. (April 14, 2015)

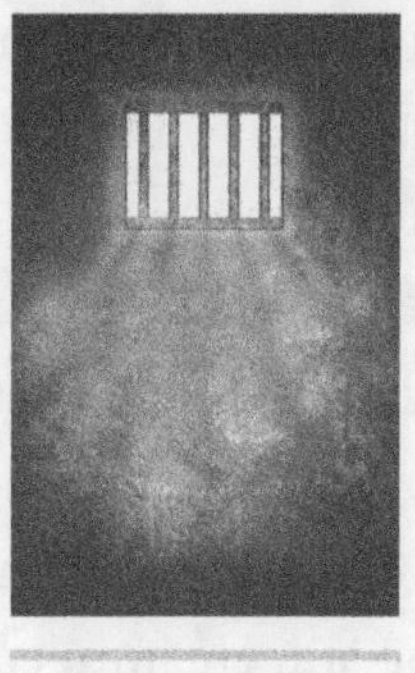

CHAPTER 10

CASE HISTORIES

CASE ONE

A lawsuit claimed that a psychiatrist failed to acknowledge suicidal behaviors of an inmate who had jumped from a height during previous detentions and failed to provide appropriate input regarding housing decision to correctional officers.

A thirty-five-year-old Caucasian male with a diagnosis of paranoid schizophrenia was booked into a large urban jail on a charge of arson. During this current detention, he showed severe psychiatric symptoms of delusions, hallucinations, mood instability, bizarre behaviors, and poor contact with reality. He had a history of multiple psychiatric hospitalizations and involuntary commitments.

Several years before his current booking, during two episodes of incarceration, he jumped off the top tier of the jail, attempting to kill himself. He sustained serious injuries, including the fracture of long bones and injury to the back. On both occasions, the same psychiatrist treated him. The jailors housed him in the top tier of the jail.

During his current detention also, the jailers housed him in the same top tier of the jail. He jumped off the top tier again. He again sustained multiple fractures, including the long bones in his legs, pelvis, and ankles with dislocation.

The psychiatrist knew that the detainee tended to jump from a height, but he failed to provide input to the officers who determined the inmate's housing. In other words, the psychiatrist disregarded the inmate's suicide vulnerability.

After I was deposed, this case settled out of court.

CASE TWO

In this case, the suit alleged that an emergency room medical staff was medically negligent, and a local jail failed to recognize imminent suicide risk and failed to provide appropriate protection to a detainee.

The police intercepted a thirty-five-year-old Caucasian male on his way to a river with his six-year-old son in his car in an apparent attempt to drive his car into the river, possibly to commit murder-suicide. He was extremely agitated, yelling and screaming, and out of control. He repeatedly demanded that the officer let him go. He made several moves to run from the police. Also, he banged his head on the ground several times. He was arrested and taken to a local ER. He told the police that he was not depressed and not on any medication or drugs. He was unemployed and supporting his family on a welfare check.

At the ER, he was emotionally labile and agitated, though he denied depression, suicidal ideation, current use of drugs, medication use, and history of mental health services. His judgment and impulse control were impaired, his mood was anxious, and his thought process was linear but logical. The ER medical staff diagnosed him with a mood disorder.

Following medical clearance, he was detained in a jail. Although the arresting officer felt the inmate was suicidal, he was not placed under suicide observation. During an early morning, the shift supervisor heard a thud from the inmate's cell wall. When checked, the inmate asked the officer to use the telephone. The officer granted his request. After exiting the cell, the inmate ran at a high speed in the hallway and hit his head with full force on a concrete wall, causing a four-inch laceration to the top of his skull. He was agitated and could not be calmed down. He was handcuffed and transported to a local hospital because he became lethargic. Later, he became unresponsive and died.

In this case, the ER medical staff accepted his denial of suicidal ideation as the basis for their decision that he was not suicidal, thereby clearing him for his detention at the county jail.

At the jail, he remained at imminent suicide risk as indicated by his continued agitation and attempt to self-harm by hitting his head on the floor and wall. The shift supervisor failed to recognize his imminent risk of suicide when he granted the inmate's request to use the phone, letting him out of the cell.

After I was deposed, the case settled out of court.

CASE THREE

Estate of Kempf v. Washington City, No. CV.15-1125, 2018 WL4354547.

Mr. Kempf, a thirty-two-year-old male, was booked in a county jail on a charge of burglary. Just before his arrest, he crashed his vehicle. The booking officer felt that he was suicidal and, therefore, placed him on suicide watch.

The next day, the jail psychiatrist diagnosed him with opioid dependence and history of depressive disorder but removed him from suicide watch without a proper suicide risk assessment. He ordered an antidepressant and an antipsychotic and scheduled to see Kempf in twelve weeks.

This man's immediate past psychiatric history indicated that he was admitted to an inpatient unit three days before his detention for suicidal ideation with a plan to "shoot himself with heroin" to kill himself. During hospitalization, he had acute heroin withdrawal symptoms, which were treated symptomatically. He was discharged from the inpatient unit with psychiatric medications, which he did not fill. His opioid dependence relapsed during the time between his discharge from the hospital and his arrest. He disclosed to the booking officer that he was recently hospitalized and that he was suicidal.

His records were not requested from his recent hospitalization. During a hearing after his arrest, he asked the judge for assistance for drug dependency and withdrawal. The judge directed the County to provide services for substance abuse. During Kempf's detention, he was placed in solitary confinement in restricted housing for a minor infraction. During the opioid withdrawal period, he hanged himself using a bedsheet, which he anchored to the cell door. During his solitary confinement, the jailers did not monitor him as required to manage inmates in restricted housing status.

In my expert report, I opined that he was at imminent risk for suicide during his detention based on drug withdrawal, suicide plan during the hospitalization three days before his detention, and his depression. I further opined that the abrupt discontinuation of suicide watch without a suicide risk assessment was a gross disregard of his medical and psychiatric need, (i.e., suicide vulnerability).

The defendant psychiatrist filed a motion for summary judgment, arguing that Kempf had no "particular vulnerability" to suicide and that the psychiatrist acted "without deliberate indifference" to his serious medical need.

The court reviewed his history, and weighed the opinions by defense and plaintiff experts, citing that "medical expert testimony is properly considered for the purpose of summary judgment in the context of §1983 deliberate indifference claims." The court cited in its opinion, *Palakovic v. Wetzel*, 854 F.3d at 223–24; see *Tatsch-Corbin v. Feathers*, 561 F. Supp. 2d. 538, 543–44 (WD Pa. 2008) (quoting *Colburn II*, 946 F.2d at 1023).

The court denied the motion for summary judgment and opined that "particular vulnerability" to suicide is determined by a combination of four factors: 1) suicidal ideation; 2) actual suicidal plan; 3) withdrawal from alcohol and drugs; and 4) a recent suicide attempt (excessive use of heroin and motor vehicle crash). The court took notice of the lengthy time between the first psychiatric visit and the scheduled visit twelve weeks later. The court further opined that the mere presence of drug use history and the mere presence of mental illness is insufficient to support a finding of suicide vulnerability.

For a plaintiff to succeed on a §1983 claim in the context of a detention suicide, plaintiff must prove the following elements: (1) that the individual had a particular vulnerability to suicide, meaning that there was a "strong likelihood, rather than a mere possibility," that a suicide would be attempted; (2) that the prison official knew or should have known of the individual's particular vulnerability; and (3) that the official acted with reckless or deliberate indifference, meaning something beyond mere negligence, to the individual's particular vulnerability.

CASE FOUR

Miranda v. County of Lake, 900 F.3d 335 (7th Cir. 2018)

The estate of Lyvita Gomes, represented by Alfredo Miranda, sued Lake County Jail, Illinois, and medical providers including Dr. H. Singh, a consultant psychiatrist, alleging that they were medically negligent and deliberately indifferent because of failure to determine Ms. Gomes's potential suicide risk.

Ms. Gomes, originally from India, was arrested for failure to appear in court on a misdemeanor charge in December 2011 and was confined to Lake County Jail. After she was booked into the jail, she began starving herself, not wanting to eat, drink, or speak, though she drank from a faucet when she thought she was not being observed. She showed no signs of mental illness. Furthermore, she denied any suicidal ideation and had no history of pre-existing mental disorder or history of suicide attempt. However, after she stopped eating and drinking she was placed on suicide watch and hunger strike protocol.

Dr. Singh was asked to evaluate her. Promptly upon receiving the consult request, he met with her, but she refused to speak with him. He spent considerable time observing her, gathering information from the jailers and other health-care professionals.

Dr. Singh found no evidence of any overt signs of mental illness such as abnormal behaviors including agitation, restlessness, and/or bizarre mannerisms, or any indications of hallucinations. She intentionally refused to eat, speak, and cooperate with the providers. However, he diagnosed her with Psychotic Disorder, Not Otherwise Specified. Ms. Gomes was a devout Catholic.

Ms. Gomes's physical condition deteriorated in a few days, raising concern by her medical providers as to her competency to make decisions in her best interest. Again, Dr. Singh evaluated her. He opined that, by this time, she did not have the capacity to decide regarding her health because her physical condition had deteriorated.

The internist in charge of the unit (not the internist defendant) transferred her to a local hospital, where she died two days later. It was determined that she died of dehydration and electrolyte imbalance. The manner of her death was ruled a suicide.

The United States District Court for the Northern District of Illinois dismissed the county defendants at summary judgment. The medical defendants, including Dr. Singh and the internist, proceeded to trial in 2016.

I testified in the jury trial that the psychiatrist fulfilled his responsibilities as a consultant psychiatrist: He did not intentionally disregard Ms. Gomes's potential psychiatric need, and he provided appropriate input to the internist. Also, he responded to the consult request in a timely manner.

During the proceedings, the court granted judgment as a matter of law under Federal Rule of Civil Procedure 50(a) for the medical providers on some claims. The estate prevailed to a modest degree on another claim. The jury failed to reach a unanimous verdict regarding the conduct of Dr. Singh and the internist. Therefore, part of the case resulted in a mistrial. The estate appealed.

The Court of Appeals ruled that "the district court abused its discretion by prohibiting (the) estate from pursuing argument that medical providers violated the Due Process Clause by failing to protect (the) inmate from harming herself; and the medical-care claims brought by pretrial detainees under the Fourteenth Amendment are subject only to the objective unreasonableness inquiry."

The court also concluded that the "Estate had failed to present enough evidence to reach the jury on the question (of) whether the medical defendants caused Gomes's death."

The court noted that the estate's expert witnesses testified that the doctors' failure to transfer Gomes to the hospital sooner allowed her deterioration to reach a dangerous point. Furthermore, Dr. Singh "knew that Gomes was clinically incompetent, but he took no steps to treat her even though she was endangering her life."

The court concluded that "the evidence was enough to support an inference on the jury's part that the delay in sending Gomes to the hospital resulted in her death, or at least lessened her chance of survival." Finally, the court opined that the estate was entitled to the opportunity to try its full case against the medical defendants.

The case against the medical defendants went to trial in 2019. Again, I testified for Dr. Singh. The estate's expert prevailed. The jury found the medical defendants liable for Ms. Gomes's death.

In this case, the Seventh Circuit concluded that the "medical care claims of pretrial detainees are governed by the due process clause of the Fourteenth Amendment, and that the standard is whether the defendant's actions were objectively unreasonable given the circumstances." Furthermore, "The obligation to intervene covers self-destructive behaviors up to and including suicide."

CASE FIVE

NeSmith v. County of San Diego, 15-CV-629 JLS (AGS)

Kris NeSmith, a twenty-one-year-old White male, a Marine, killed himself by hanging in his cell at Vista Detention Facility (VDF) San Diego on March 1, 2014, using a bedsheet anchored to a light fixture.

NeSmith's wife filed a lawsuit against San Diego County, California, its sheriff, and VDF, alleging causes of action under 42. U.S. C. §1983 for deliberate indifference to Mr. NeSmith's serious medical needs, failure to train, failure to implement policies, negligence, and wrongful death.

NeSmith joined the U.S. Marines in 2010. He began to experience severe mental illness after he was nearly shot in the head during training at Camp Pendleton's Horno Rifle range in April 2013. He had thoughts of suicide and hearing voices. He went AWOL (absence without leave) and married his girlfriend on June 23, 2013. During the honeymoon, he attempted suicide by using a dog leash, fearful that he would be taken back to Camp Pendleton.

NeSmith attempted suicide again by hanging himself in his closet on July 20, 2013. The sheriff took him back to Camp

Pendleton. While at the base, NeSmith erratically attacked a regiment officer. On August 6, 2013, he was taken to the brig on charges of being AWOL and assaulting a regiment officer. At the base, he attempted suicide by a cell phone charger wire, and his wife thwarted this attempt.

NeSmith was sentenced to four months in the brig, where he spent 102 days in solitary confinement. While at the brig, he attempted suicide two more times and was under constant watch and regular mental health evaluation. He was severely depressed. He was diagnosed with mixed personality disorder with borderline and antisocial features.

NeSmith was released on November 19, 2013, on appellate leave. He was malnourished and paranoid, and during that weekend he drank heavily.

On November 27, 2013, he left home, and beat up and strangled a stranger causing physical injuries to the stranger. He then returned to his home.

On November 28, 2013, he left home again at night and had an encounter with a neighbor, causing life-threatening injuries to the neighbor. He then returned to his home.

The next day in a parking lot, he attempted to strangle his wife, calling her by a different name. The sheriff was called to the domestic violence scene. Police identified NeSmith as the person involved in the offenses the previous nights. He was taken into custody and detained at VDF. He did not have a roommate. He was charged with domestic violence, attempted murder, mayhem, and resisting arrest.

During his arraignment on December 3, 2013, NeSmith knew he might be facing life in prison. He pleaded with his father to bail him out, but his father told him he could not afford a $2 million bond. NeSmith became extremely distraught and again expressed suicidal ideation, telling his father he would kill himself. His father informed various county personnel, including the district attorney, that his son had made suicidal statements.

NeSmith had his preliminary hearing on February 26, 2014.

On Saturday, March 1, 2014, at about 0658 hours, a deputy found NeSmith motionless, wedged between the toilet and the bunk with a piece of torn white sheet wrapped around his neck. He was pronounced dead at 0735 hours. The cause of his death was cited as hanging. The toxicology report showed that he did not have alcohol or drugs of abuse in his system.

The night before NeSmith hanged himself, an officer observed a makeshift noose hanging from his light fixture. The officer merely commented, "What are you doing? (Trying to) Kill yourself? Take that down." The officer did nothing further.

A medical intake at VDF on November 30, 2013, shows that the questions concerning suicidal ideation, past and current psychiatric problems, use of street drugs, use of medications, and medical and mental health history, and mental status findings were marked N (No). Interestingly, the question, "Have you ever served in the U.S. Military?" was also marked N. Following the intake, he was housed alone at VDF.

Limited medication prescription profile shows that NeSmith was on Desyrel [Trazodone] 50 mg a day on December 5, 2013, which was increased to 100 mg a week later. Prozac 20 mg a day was started on December 12, 2013, and Sinequan [Doxepin] 100 mg a day on January 9, 2014.

A mental health worker noted [qualifications unidentified] on December 4, 2013, that "his father called the DA, who then called the sergeant" to inform them that NeSmith told his father he would kill himself. This worker further noted that NeSmith denied any suicidal ideation or psychiatric history. Under the diagnosis section, it was noted "Persistent D/O and Cannabis Dependence." On December 5, 2013, an entry by a psychiatrist shows after a cursory "psych eval" that she started him on Desyrel 50 mg a day.

A note on December 10, 2013, shows that NeSmith requested to see "psych" for "PTSD and Depression."

A note on December 12, 2013, by the psychiatrist shows that NeSmith complained of sleep difficulties, depression, nightmares, and worry. On examination, she noted that he "endorsed depression" but no psychotic symptoms or mania. She did not document any self-injurious ideation. She diagnosed him with "309.81" [PTSD] and "304. 4" [Amphetamine and other stimulant dependence]. The psychiatrist started him on Prozac 20 mg a day and Prazosin 1 mg at bedtime and she increased the dose of Desyrel to 100 mg at night.

On December 23 and 24, 2013, NeSmith refused his medications by not showing up in the pill line. He reportedly asked to discontinue his medication.

On January 9, 2014, NeSmith complained of "trouble with Trazodone" because reportedly it caused an anger problem. He was again seen by the psychiatrist, who diagnosed him with primary insomnia [307.42]. She discontinued his Trazodone but started him on Doxepin 100 mg.

As of January 20, 2014, NeSmith continued to refuse Doxepin. The next day, Doxepin was discontinued.

The last time he was seen by "psych" was on February 2, 2014, for increasing anxiety, rumination that he let down his family, depression, trouble sleeping, and increasing self-isolative behaviors. He denied suicidal and homicidal ideation. He was assessed to be "not an acute risk of harm to self or others." The note further showed "no indication for inpatient hospitalization or placement on 5150."

I opined in my report and during deposition that Kris NeSmith posed significant suicide risk during his detention at VDF, given the history of multiple suicide attempts since May 2013.

NeSmith's suicide risk remained high throughout his confinement at VDF, despite his denial of suicidal ideation. Off and on he refused his medications and isolated himself in the jail. He was anxious, agitated, and ruminated on "letting down his family." He had significant problem with sleep, which was interrupted by nightmares.

NeSmith had significant prior mental health history including depressive disorder, possibly PTSD, and substance abuse, including methamphetamine and marijuana.

VDF should have known that NeSmith was of substantial suicide risk but placed him in the general population during his confinement instead of a suicide-resistant special cell. He specifically expressed a strong wish to die once he realized that he was facing a long sentence, possibly a life sentence. Also, he felt hopeless and distraught when his father told him that he could not afford a $2 million bond. He refused all treatment after January 21, 2014. He refused to eat and began to isolate himself during the weekend—yet another indicator of suicide risk.

The officer who saw him with a noose the night before did nothing except to comment, "What are you doing. Kill yourself?

Take it down." The officer had the duty to place NeSmith on suicide watch immediately and inform the mental health staff. His failure to take the inmate's suicidal behavior was a reckless disregard of his serious psychiatric/medical need.

The care, skill, and knowledge exercised or exhibited by jail officials during the incarceration of NeSmith at the San Diego County Jail from November 2013 to March 2014 were substantially below the acceptable professional standards and care, and such conduct was a cause of bringing harm to NeSmith.

I concluded that the VDF jail staff knew that Mr. NeSmith was of obvious and substantial risk the night before his suicide and serious medical need by failing to take appropriate and necessary action. County officials also ignored NeSmith's risk, even after his father spoke with county officials. These failures directly caused and/or contributed to his suicidal death on March 1, 2014.

San Diego County and deputies moved for summary judgment. In denying the summary judgment the court noted that plaintiff expert, Dr. Daniel, had criticized the County's intake process. "All the county did was going through the ten intake questions in a cursory manner and taking 'no' for an answer to question on suicidal ideation is a significant flaw in the execution of a comprehensive suicide prevention program in a jail setting" because "many seriously suicidal inmates hide their true intent to harm (the)msel(ves). It is the role of the custodial and mental health staff to consider all the factors in determining the risk of given inmate."

The court noted that Dr. Daniel concluded that Mr. NeSmith "posed a significant risk at the time he was booked and placed in the custody of VDF, given the history of multiple suicide attempts since May 2013 and that VDF should have known that he was a substantial suicide risk." And "According to Dr. Daniel there were several factors that should have placed the jail on notice that Mr. NeSmith 'had a significant suicide risk at the time he was booked' including 'his young age, he is White. He is basically coming to the jail the first time and having to face a violent offense charge.'" Based on these factors, the prison "should have . . . documented" the risk and "alerted the staff (as to) the possibility of (a) potential suicide."

Regarding the suicide prevention policy at the jail, the court recognized Dr. Daniel's opinion that it "offers no guidance on identifying inmates who would be potentially suicidal . . . Also, the jail policy does not address different levels of suicide watch."

CASE SIX

In the United States District Court, Eastern District of Wisconsin: Case No.:18-CV-896

The estate of Ruth Freiwald, who committed suicide, filed a deliberate indifference lawsuit against Adeyemi Fatoki, MD, the jail psychiatrist claiming that he abruptly discontinued her Klonopin and Gabapentin, which caused her suicide. I testified for the defense of the psychiatrist. The jury returned a verdict for him.

Ms. Freiwald, a fifty-one-year-old White female, a detainee at the Work Release Center (also known as Huber Center), of Brown County Jail, Wisconsin, left the center at 6:30 a.m. on November 2, 2016, for class at a local training center. She stepped in front of a moving vehicle, sustaining severe injuries. She died on November 6, 2016, at a local hospital. The manner of her death was ruled a suicide and the immediate cause of death as blunt trauma to her torso and extremities.

In October 2016, Ms. Freiwald was sentenced to two years of probation with 45 days in jail with Huber privileges, on a charge of Operating While Intoxicated (OWI). Previously, on February 8, 2016, she attempted suicide while driving under the influence of an unknown quantity of Klonopin by pulling her vehicle into traffic and was hit by a truck. She was an unbelted driver.

After the February 2016 incident, she received mental health treatment for depression, anxiety, and PTSD by local providers including psychiatrists, therapists, and nurse practitioners. As of October 2016, she was on Prozac 20 mg a day, Gabapentin 600 mg a day, Lisinopril 20 mg a day, Klonopin 1 mg daily (plus 0.5 mg as needed), and Diclofenac 75 mg twice a day. The sentencing judge ordered her to take all prescribed medications, maintain sobriety, and provide information regarding her medications to the jail staff.

Ms. Freiwald voluntarily reported to the Brown County Jail at about 7:18 p.m. on October 27, 2016. She did not bring her prescribed medications with her to jail. After the intake and booking procedure was completed at the main facility, she reported to the Huber Center. The next day, at her request, her son brought her medications to the main jail. Based on the information provided by her, the booking officer determined that she was not at suicide risk.

On October 29, 2016, a nurse contacted Dr. Fatoki by telephone. Dr. Fatoki approved Prozac, Lisinopril, and Diclofenac. Dr. Fatoki did not have enough information regarding Gabapentin and Klonopin; therefore, he ordered a Release of Information (ROI) to obtain the needed information. He also ordered the inmate to be observed for any withdrawal symptoms.

A Medical Services Request filed by the inmate on October 30, 2016, indicated that her "blood pressure was so high that I have a migraine headache. I am having a hard time thinking straight. I am having four exams this week. I have to be able to think clearly."

Ms. Freiwald expected that she would be placed on electronic monitoring and that her jail stay would be limited to one or two days. Officers at the Huber Center had not observed her having any withdrawal symptoms. Instead, they described her as calm.

On the morning of November 2, 2016, she texted a family member that "I did not expect these set of circumstances." She was upset about having to stay in jail for the entire 45 days, contrary to her expectation that she would spend only the weekend and be on house arrest. She described her situation in the jail as "hard, food was terrible, TV was on all the time—I could not sleep." She sent an email to a friend at 7:42 a.m. on November 2, 2016, with the message "no way out."

I opined in my report and deposition that she was not a suicide risk when she entered the Brown County Jail on October 27, 2016, though she was anxious about going to jail. She did not have any observed withdrawal symptoms from Klonopin and Gabapentin. Observations of and interactions by officers showed that she was not agitated, depressed, tearful, or hopeless, but she was looking forward to attending school. The medical services request filed by her did not show any indicators of self-harm because she was mostly concerned about her blood pressure medication and headache. On the October 30, 2016, her thoughts were forward-looking in that she planned to take the "four exams this week." Her family members did not think that she was suicidal either.

She showed no withdrawal symptoms from Klonopin or Gabapentin during her stay at the Huber Center. Except for headache, most likely due to not taking her Lisinopril, she did not have, either by self-report or observation by officers, any physical withdrawal symptoms such as nausea, vomiting, abdominal pain, or excessive sweating and tremors. Also, she had no psychological symptoms of withdrawal—except for anxiety, which is related to her having to stay for the entire 45 days of her sentence.

I opined that Dr. Fatoki did not deviate from the standard of care in approving Lisinopril, Diclofenac, and Fluoxetine and not approving Klonopin and Gabapentin on October 29, 2016. He made his decision to manage her medications based on the information he received from the nurse. It is a standard practice to "bridge" an inmate's medication based on information received from a unit nurse. Gathering additional information is standard clinical procedure. Klonopin and Gabapentin were not among the no-miss medications such as insulin, blood thinners, or similar medications where missing a dose would harm a patient.

Dr. Fatoki's decision not to taper the dose of Klonopin fell within standard of care because the dose of Klonopin that the inmate was taking was well below the daily dose of a benzodiazepine requiring tapering to avoid symptoms such as seizures, tremor, and serious psychiatric symptoms. Klonopin 1 mg daily is considered a low daily dose. It is a common practice in jails and prisons for physicians not to prescribe benzodiazepines for a variety of reasons, including bartering the medications for other favors.

The direct examination by the defense attorney was limited to four areas of inquiry:

1. Was "not renewing" Klonopin 1 mg for a jail inmate appropriate?
2. Did she have any withdrawal symptoms; more specifically did she have any suicidal ideation or behaviors because of non-renewal of Klonopin?
3. Plausible explanations of why she took her life?
4. Did Dr. Fatoki exercise appropriate professional judgment when he did not renew the inmate's Klonopin?

The plaintiff's attorney mostly concentrated on her lengthy history of mental illness and past suicide attempt and her history of Klonopin use. He challenged my opinions on lack of peer-reviewed articles that support abrupt discontinuation of Klonopin.

Suicidal thoughts as a withdrawal symptom of benzodiazepine are extremely rare, even if the discontinuation of high dose of Klonopin is abrupt. The FDA literature on Klonopin does not mention it (www.accessdata.fda.gov).

The peak time for withdrawal symptoms from benzodiazepine is about 2 weeks from the date of cessation. Rebound anxiety, experienced by some patients, occurs around 7 to 14 days.

When faced with life's difficulties, Ms. Freiwald showed a pattern of suicidal statements and behaviors. Before her suicide attempt on February 8, 2016, she faced a business and financial loss, which was cited as the main reason for her suicide attempt. In the mid-1980s, when she was in college, she reportedly expressed suicidal ideation. Finally, she expressed intense displeasure for being in jail and was upset that she must serve 45 days.

CASE HISTORIES BY RICHARD LICHTEN, JAIL AND POLICE EXPERT

Richard Lichten presents case histories 7, 8, and 9 to demonstrate what can happen when the correctional staff fails to follow established suicide prevention policies and procedures.

CASE SEVEN

A twenty-three-year-old male was incarcerated at a jail from June 27, 2014 to September 27, 2014, for a domestic violence charge. On September 27, 2014, he was discovered hanging in his cell. He was taken down, CPR was administered, and he was sent to a hospital. He died on October 20, 2014.

The decedent's family filed a lawsuit against the county law enforcement agency. It claimed he was improperly housed and did not receive proper mental health treatment.

The plaintiffs alleged that the inmate had a history of mental illness and suicide attempts. A licensed mental health clinician at intake noted that his reported history of suicide attempts was "questionable" and "appeared exaggerated and fabricated" and his "insight questionable."

On July 5, 2014, he was allegedly insubordinate because he stated he was suicidal, and when the jail personnel would not take his threats seriously, he used profanity and was disrespectful toward the staff. He also threatened to fight the staff if he was sent to the discipline cell. However, he was ordered to serve time in the discipline cell for his disruptive behavior. The discipline report showed that the mental health staff saw him and advised that he could be housed in a discipline cell.

The jail records show that on July 5, 2014, mental health staff evaluated him. During the evaluation, he reportedly threatened to bang his head against the wall or glass in the cell. He was reported to have stated to the mental health staff that he needed help. However, the staff determined that he was not psychotic but did have "antisocial personality traits." He was also determined to be hoarding medications and "engaging in other maladaptive behaviors."

The records further show that on July 6, 2014, he reported he had swallowed two razors because he wanted to kill himself. On September 8, 2014, he reported he was feeling suicidal and that he had made prior suicide attempts. On September 22, 2014, he was recorded by jail personnel as saying he had made a recent suicide attempt.

The jail movement records show that he was on suicide watch on September 25, 2014 and was moved to a discipline cell on September 27, 2014. About five hours and twenty-six minutes after he was placed in a discipline cell, an officer found him hanging from a noose made of cloth, anchored to a damaged light fixture.

The plaintiffs alleged that the jail records show that a psychiatrist was made aware of the decedent's suicidal ideation on September 25, 2014, however, he was not seen by a psychiatrist.

The jail records show that the required 30-minute safety cell check of his discipline cell was conducted 31 minutes late, and it was not conducted properly. The video evidence shows the officer walking down the middle of the hallway, looking down at a paper in his hand. The officer never glanced inside the cells, including the decedent's cell, as he quickly walked right by. This same officer falsified the cell check log by stating the check was, indeed, performed. His discipline cell was not searched for contraband before the inmate was placed in the cell.

After analysis and study of the case, I opined that the officer in charge deviated from the standard of care by not performing the inmate safety check on September 27, 2014. Furthermore, the officer falsified the safety check log.

In addition, the officer deviated from the standard of care when the decedent told the officer that he did not speak with the psychiatrist over the past few days about feeling suicidal, and the officer took no action to investigate this claim.

The officer knew the decedent was suicidal on September 27, 2014, and knew he had just been transferred back to the discipline cell from being on suicide watch.

The officer showed a conscious disregard of the decedent's safety by not acting to mitigate his suicide risk. Jail policy stated: "Any expression of suicidal actions or thought, or any talk of suicide, should be brought to the immediate attention of a supervisor and to Medical and Mental Health staff." This was not done. The officer did nothing other than tell the decedent to stop kicking the discipline cell door.

Had the cell been routinely and properly searched, the noose may have been discovered before it was used.

Additionally, the damaged light fixture may have been found and repaired. The decedent had anchored his noose on this light fixture.

After I submitted the report, the county settled the case.

When an inmate tells a correctional officer that he or she is suicidal, the correctional officer must take swift and proper action. The officer must remove the inmate from the housing unit and place him/her on suicide watch and refer to a mental health professional. The officer must document the incident.

When correctional officers conduct the required inmate safety/welfare checks, they must remember the reasons for these checks. The reasons include (1) to ensure the inmate is not in medical distress, and (2) to ensure the inmate is not involved in criminality (making weapons, involved in a fight, etc.). To perform a proper check, the correctional officer must stop in front of the cell and look inside at the inmate long enough to determine if all is well. This can take several seconds to several minutes. To recap, in this case the correctional officer walked right by the inmate's cell without looking in the cell while the inmate was hanging by his neck.

Correctional officers must search the inmates' property and inspect the housing area often for dangerous conditions. In this case, had the inmate's property been searched there was a chance the correctional officers may have found the ligature the inmate later used and may have observed the damaged light which enabled the inmate to anchor his ligature for hanging.

As the jail practices expert, I did not opine on the actions of the mental health providers.

CASE EIGHT

The mother of a forty-four-year-old jail inmate who hanged himself sued a county law enforcement agency, claiming that he was improperly housed and did not receive proper mental health treatment.

The plaintiff alleged that during the evening hours on September 24, 2015, her son swallowed a full bottle (60 pills) of Klonopin in a suicide attempt at her home. The plaintiff called for his brother to come to the home to help. Once the brother arrived, a struggle ensued between the brother and the decedent. The family summoned law enforcement personnel.

The plaintiff further alleged the decedent's brother told the dispatcher about his suicide attempts and his history of mental illness.

When the deputies arrived at the home (the plaintiff alleged) the decedent's brother told the deputies of his suicide attempt by overdose. The deputies then arrested him for assaulting his brother. He was taken to the local hospital for medical clearance (not mental health clearance). Once he was medically cleared, he was booked into the jail.

On the night of September 27, 2015, he was found hanging in his cell in the Administrative Segregation unit. He used a bedsheet as a noose and anchored the other end to the cell's air vent.

The plaintiff alleged the decedent had gone three days without his needed medications and without being seen by a psychiatrist. She further alleged the jail staff and the medical and mental health staff knew of his past suicide attempts and that they showed "deliberate indifference" to the decedent's serious medical and mental health needs.

After analyzing all the evidence, I opined that the arresting officers knew that he intentionally ingested dozens of prescription medication pills at his home. They failed to recognize his behaviors and actions of taking the pills that were indicative of and consistent with a suicide attempt. They also failed to inform the hospital ER staff that he had ingested the numerous pills, thereby not conforming to their professional responsibility to inform the ER staff of this critical information.

Not advising the ER staff of his suicide attempt by overdose was below the standard of care and was unreasonable. Had the ER staff been told that he had taken the pills, their decision to release him to the jail might have been different.

I further opined that the deputy in the jail's classification unit failed to follow established policy and wrongly classified and housed the decedent in Administrative Segregation instead on suicide watch in a high observation unit. To make matters worse, when the decedent was wrongly placed in his cell in Administrative Segregation, he was also given a bedsheet. The policy states the decedent should have been given a safety garment and blanket. The decedent hanged himself with the issued bedsheet.

I opined that housing a suicidal inmate alone in Administrative Segregation with a bedsheet and without closely observing/monitoring the known suicidal inmate showed a conscious disregard for his safety.

The evidence showed that the nursing staff and the jail watch commander failed to follow the jail's well-established suicide prevention policy. Had the suicide prevention policy (as well as the classification training manual) been followed, the decedent would not have been placed in Administrative

Segregation. Instead, he would have been properly housed in the Enhanced Observation Housing (next to the nursing station) on suicide watch.

After I submitted my report, the defense counsel deposed me. During the deposition, the attorney spent considerable time questioning me about the jail policies and procedures and staff training on classification and housing of mentally ill suicidal inmates. I explained that the jail's classification policies and procedures were well written and easy to understand but were not followed. I testified that the actions of the deputies were inconsistent with their training. If the policies and procedures were adhered to and had the deputies acted consistent with their training, the decedent would not have been able to hang himself.

After my deposition, the county settled the case.

The takeaway in this case is that no matter how good and clear the jail's policy and procedures may be and no matter how well trained the correctional staff may be, if the correctional staff fail to follow their policies and procedures and fail to follow their training, it is all meaningless.

CASE NINE

Pulera v. Sarzant, 966 F.3d 540, 556 (7th Cir. 2020)

In this case, I was retained by the defense. An adult male inmate who attempted suicide by hanging in his cell sued the county law enforcement officials.

Mr. Pulera was arrested on April 21, 2012, for felony bail jumping and for violating the conditions of his bond by drinking alcohol. He was then taken to and booked at the Kenosha County Jail.

Mr. Pulera alleged that during booking he exhibited signs of severe depression, distress, and self-harm tendencies. The medical/mental health screening questionnaires were completed as part of the intake and booking process. He reported that he was prescribed Clonazepam for anxiety and Tramadol for pain.

He alleged that he was not placed on suicide watch and that no medical or mental health professional was called to see him, that he was incorrectly housed in a general population cell, and that his cell assignment was "deliberately indifferent" to his safety because during the intake and booking process he yelled suicidal statements.

On April 23, 2012, at about 0140 hours, he attached one end of his bedsheet to his upper cell bars, made a noose out of the other end, and hanged. Within minutes, officers acted to release him from the noose. He was admitted to an intensive care unit. He survived.

Mr. Pulera alleged the defendants were slow to come to his aid. The medical help and the call to the Fire Department were allegedly delayed until after he was taken down.

After a thorough analysis of all the evidence in this case, I opined that Mr. Pulera did not exhibit suicidal cues during his arrest, intake, and booking, or while housed in his general population cell up until the moment he attempted to hang himself. This evidence includes his statements that he was not suicidal on the following jail intake forms: He answered "no" to the questions on each form regarding suicidal ideation.

1. The Transporting Officer Observation Report

2. The Medical/Mental Screening Visual Observation Report
3. The Zone One Protective Holding Report
4. The Medical/Mental Screening Form
5. The Mental Health Risk Assessment Form
6. The Medical/Mental Screening Medical Questionnaire

Further, based on the evidence, I opined that the intake and booking staff and/or housing correctional officers did not know (or ignored) a risk/threat or act in an improper, uncaring manner, or fail to exercise reasonable care during Mr. Pulera's intake.

Mr. Pulera was properly classified and housed in the general population. When the corrections officers discovered him hanging in his cell, they acted within two minutes and saved his life. There was no delay in rescue.

I further opined that Mr. Pulera was not detained under conditions posing a substantial risk of serious harm.

Intake and booking staff had no reason to believe he was a suicide risk. Also, the jail's intake and booking procedures were followed at intake. The jail had sufficient suicide prevention intake screening procedures in place. The jail also properly trained the correctional staff in suicide prevention. I opined that policies or training, or lack thereof were not the "moving force" for his suicide attempt.

The defendant officers filed for a summary judgment. In granting the summary judgment, the district court concluded that "There was no genuine dispute that all officials responded reasonably to the information each had."

The plaintiff appealed the district court decision to the Seventh Circuit Court of Appeals. The Seventh Circuit opined that "Under the totality of the chaotic circumstances, the officers' swift actions were indisputably reasonable and preclude a finding that they violated Pulera's constitutional rights. It is unfortunate that Pulera attempted to kill himself and fortunate that he did not succeed. That a tragedy almost happened under the watch of jail officers, though, does not mean the officers are responsible. All that one can expect—and all the Constitution demands—is that officials respond reasonably to the situation. Because there is no genuine dispute that all the defendants here did so, we AFFIRM the judgment of the district court."

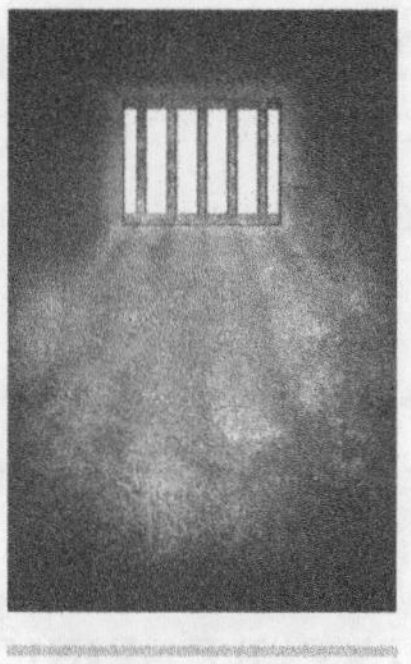

CHAPTER 11

ATTORNEYS
ON EXPERTS

The fundamental role of the expert is to educate the jury on scientific or technical matters relevant to the case. His/her role is to teach and persuade the layperson jury to understand the issues and facts to decide the case and reach a verdict. In a correctional lawsuit, the jury will ultimately decide whether a correctional health-care professional deviated from the standard of care and exercised appropriate professional judgment in mitigating the suicide risk of an inmate. Similarly, the jury will decide if the correctional official disregarded the inmate's serious medical need, thus causing or contributing to severe injury or suicide.

But it's more than just expert testimony in play concerning the evaluation of claims. Some attorneys rely on consulting experts (those not designated to give expert testimony) to give them case-specific advice. For instance, an attorney may rely on expert consultants' opinions concerning his/her client's conduct—a frank discussion of strengths and weaknesses of tactical options and factual and legal positions. Also, the attorney may employ consulting experts to assist with preparation for the deposition of opposing expert witnesses and sometimes to vet the testifying witnesses' opinions.

RULES GOVERNING EXPERT OPINIONS

Historically, the basis of expert testimony originated with the Frye Test in 1923. (*Frye v. the United States*, 293 F. 1013, (DC Circuit 1923). In this case, an expert witness was not allowed to testify regarding a lie detector test (systolic blood pressure deception test) because the test had "not yet gained such standing and scientific recognition among physiological and psychological authorities." However, this case paved the way for establishing the standard of general acceptance theory for expert testimony. This standard was replaced with Federal Rules of Evidence 702, 703, and 705.

Rule 702 states that an expert may testify if:

(a) the expert's scientific, technical, or other specialized knowledge will help the trier of fact to understand the evidence or to determine a fact in issue;

(b) the testimony is based on sufficient facts or data;

(c) the testimony is the product of reliable principles and methods; and

(d) the expert has reliably applied the principles and methods to the facts of the case.

Rule 703 states: "An expert may base an opinion on facts or data in the case that the expert has been made aware of or personally observed. If experts in the particular field would reasonably rely on those kinds of facts or data in forming an opinion on the subject, they need not be admissible for the opinion to be admitted. But if the facts or data would otherwise be inadmissible, the proponent of the opinion may disclose them to the jury only if their probative value in helping the jury evaluate the opinion substantially outweighs their prejudicial effect."

Rule 705 states: "Unless the court orders otherwise, an expert may state an opinion—and give the reasons for it—without first testifying to the underlying facts or data. But the expert may be required to disclose those facts or data on cross-examination."

The courts have explained Rule 702 in the context of scientific expert testimony by laying out the following nonexclusive factors:

(1) Whether the theory or technique in question has been or can be tested

(2) Whether the theory or technique has been subjected to peer review and publication

(3) The known or potential rate of error of the theory or technique and whether means exist for controlling its operation

(4) The extent to which the theory or technique has been accepted

The first factor [702(a)] generally requires the expert witness's special knowledge to be helpful in/relevant to the case. Rule 702(b) ensures the expert's opinion isn't just his "ipse dixit"—(i.e., "It is so because I'm a super-smart expert, and I say it is so)." It must have a basis. The third and fourth factors [702(c)-(d)] require a credible relationship between the facts/data and the conclusion (i.e., the principles and methods used by the expert must be reliably used by experts in the same field), as well as assurance that the expert correctly applied them. In scientific cases, this last 702 factor focuses on replicability.

The weight given to any of the 702 factors, and even which factors apply, depends on the issues being litigated. The first must always apply, but sometimes none of the others do. For instance, some expert witnesses give non-scientific expert opinions about things as diverse as "How does a reasonable construction worker use a jackhammer?" And "What is the reasonable cost of an MRI?"

State courts have by and large relied upon the federal rules with slight variations. For instance, the Texas Supreme Court stipulated the following rules:

(1) The extent to which the theory has been or can be tested

(2) The extent to which the technique relies upon the subjective interpretation of the expert

(3) Whether the theory has been subjected to peer review and/or publication

(4)   The technique's potential rate of error

(5)   Whether the underlying theory or technique has been generally accepted as valid by the relevant scientific community

(6)   The non-judicial uses that have been made of the theory or technique

Because it's unlikely that a juror can ever be educated to such a level that he or she is capable of individually assessing a health-care provider's actions, the role of the expert in the real-world practice of law has evolved to cover both establishing the standard (a legal matter usually supplied by the judge) and providing an opinion whether the facts available to him or her suggest the standard was/was not met (the role of the fact-finder—the jurors). This curious blending of principles results in jurors often deciding cases by reference to which expert they choose to believe if the experts differ in their conclusions.

ATTORNEYS' OPINIONS ON EXPERTS

I sought opinions from thirty-six attorneys involved in suicide-related lawsuits in the United States on their hiring practice of experts. Twenty-five attorneys responded: twenty in writing (nineteen agreed to use their names and one remained anonymous) and five verbally. (Their narratives are included in Appendix 4.)

Questions:

1.   Considering Rule 702, what factors do you weigh in choosing an expert to work on your case?

2. Are any or all factors noted in Rule 702, or any other factors given special weight?

Attorney responses show several important considerations besides emphasizing the general requirements consistent with Rule 702.

Desirable Attributes of an Expert

Attorneys look for experts who are knowledgeable, credible, relatable, persuasive, and with good communication skills. Knowledge of the subject matter of the lawsuit is the primary requisite of an expert. Peer-reviewed publications, general acceptance of his/her theories and methodology by other experts, and teaching responsibilities generally determine an expert's knowledge and expertise. More specifically, publications on correctional mental health, correctional practices, and suicide will set the expert apart from others.

Even if the expert is highly knowledgeable on correctional practices and suicide-related issues, their knowledge does not mean much if the jury does not believe him/her. The jury determines the credibility of an expert in several dimensions. These include knowledge, trustworthiness, relatability, confidence, and humility.

Arrogance generally turns the jury away. Attorney Christopher Grabarek stated: "Arrogance is an indicator that the expert will not be likable or understandable. Their inflated ego encourages them to believe that the jurors should be honored to be in their presence." Attorney Jesus Eduardo Arias opined that: "With inherent authority on the field by way of his experience, but with the humble ability (the expert should be able) to talk to the jury not in a condescending manner, but rather in an explanatory manner."

Reliability of opinions is shown only where the testimony is based on sufficient facts or data and is the product of generally accepted principles and methods. As scientific knowledge evolves, an expert who opines with absolute certainty is generally not well accepted. Experts must be authentic and not slick, fudge facts, or commit a series of minor errors in data analysis.

Choosing an Expert

The selection of an expert is case-specific. It can be the most important decision an attorney makes in a case if the attorney feels expert testimony will be of benefit.

Attorneys Patrick Provenzale, Robin Frazer Clark, Herbert Terrell, and Marlon Primes consider and weigh a potential expert's diversity of professional qualifications, including academic, practical, and research credentials and peer-reviewed articles' authorship. In addition, experience in testifying for both the plaintiff and defendant or qualified by a court of law to testify is preferable.

Attorney Eric Frederickson stated that a U.S. appellate court qualifying an expert is a great asset. Frazer reported that: "You will want to make sure you have that opinion (qualifying by an appellate court) as often. Many courts need only for another court already to have ruled on the expert's qualifications in a particular field for the current court to bless the expert. You will also want to obtain as many orders denying Daubert motions on the expert by trial judges as possible. What other trial judges have done on Daubert motions on the expert is very persuasive to most sitting trial judges. It not only makes their job easier but also gives them confidence in ruling that the expert may testify."

Attorney Amy Boring stated: "First, I take a good look at the specific facts of the case and determine what it is that I need the expert to discuss or clarify. Some of the things I look for include area of expertise, length of practice, publications, experience in litigation, and current employment. These factors help narrow the field of potential experts."

Attorney Amanda Bridson stated: "If other courts had found an expert's opinions to be based on sound methods and reasoning, I feel good about my ability to withstand future Daubert challenges."

An attorney summarized his position as follows: "I look for experts whose credibility is demonstrated by their history of providing opinions for both sides of a contested issue. Sometimes that is not possible because the expert has never been retained in a case where he could have offered such an opinion. Still, the expert must at least be willing to concede that, for instance, a doctor really could breach a standard of care by perforating an artery during a cardiac catheterization procedure and then, if appropriate, be able to explain in his lawsuit why he didn't. This shows reasonableness of thought that enhances credibility."

The attorney further commented that he looks for experts who are, in fact, experts. He does not want an expert who "becomes" an expert (for instance, through study after being retained) specifically to give testimony in a particular case on a particular topic. He looks for an expert who is already an expert in his or her field. Indeed, research conducted, and opinions generated solely for the purpose of litigation should be excluded. The expert must have been studying the subject matter for some time. The expert must tell the attorney that his/her case is a "dog when his case is a dog."

But ultimately, the attorney is a litigator, with the job of presenting the best case for his or her clients. They must be concerned with the persuasive presentation of the case as much as the legal and factual side of things. Assuming excellent competence, credentials, and actual field expertise, the attorney needs an expert witness whose testimony is likely to persuade a jury to adopt the attorney's opinions. The expert becomes the attorney's teammate for winning the case. Credentials are important, but so is authenticity.

Pragmatically, in the context of a case, attorneys see one of their jobs as convincing the court to give special weight to the factors least favorable to their opponent's expert's testimony when trying to exclude a witness and his/her opinions. Thus, when defending against the opponent's motion to exclude an expert, attorneys emphasize the factor on which his/her expert is strongest and try to explain why the others are not applicable. Generally, courts are predisposed to allow expert testimony rather than exclude it.

Regarding bias, Attorney Primes stated: "I do not ever want to be associated with an expert who may be perceived as a hired gun. So an expert that has experience testifying for plaintiffs and defendants is very valuable. In litigation, there are often competing experts, and you want the finder of fact to give your expert the benefit of the doubt because of their reputation for being even-handed and practical. If the expert has set guidelines for formulating his opinions, they should be applied equally to plaintiffs and defendants."

It is important to note any state-specific requirements that may have been adopted for expert witness testimony. Some states have specific rules governing a testifying expert, so it is important to ensure that the expert meets these requirements before proceeding.

Knowledge of Law and Experience

Experts must know and be familiar with the law, including the statutes and administrative codes related to the issue at hand. Attorney Kathleen Griffith stated: "Most jail suicide cases involve §1983 civil rights claim which can be complex and convoluted. One of the factors is the expert's ability to handle difficult questions during a deposition. If an expert has a difficult time explaining or supporting his findings in a deposition, then chances are he will not present well as a witness during the trial."

Attorney Bridson emphasized "particularized" education, training, or experience that closely aligns with the issues in the case. An expert could help the jury understand the unique demands that incarceration can have on a person's mental health and how a prison can and should respond to a prisoner experiencing a mental health crisis.

Attorney Frazer noted: "The most important factor is the amount of actual hands-on experience an expert has in the subject field. You need an expert who has practiced or supervised staff in a correctional setting to be able to rebut that argument through an affidavit or deposition testimony."

Attorney Primes stated: "The expert's resume and background should indicate that he or she has an excellent knowledge and mastery of their field of study."

Attorney Frederickson noted: "Similar situations to those involved in my case, the better. At the least, the expert must have experience treating patients with similar mental health needs to the suicide victim in my case. It is highly preferable, though not required, that the expert have experience working in a correctional facility or otherwise treating incarcerated patients."

Attorney Christopher Morris commented, "First, I like my expert to be a practitioner in the field at issue. The jury often views experts that have long since removed themselves from the day-to-day activities as simply a 'hired gun.'"

Consultant Anita Korwin noted that: "When reviewing a case about suicide of an incarcerated individual, it is important that the expert understands the unique challenges that can be encountered in the correctional setting."

Ability to Support Opinions with Facts and Evidence

To ensure that the testimony is based on sufficient facts or data, experts must be prepared to point to the specific evidence in the case (medical records, jail/prison records, fact witness testimony, and other documents) on which their opinions are based. Regarding reliable principles and methods, Frederickson stated that experts should be able to show that the way they have analyzed the case is in line with methods generally used in their field. It is helpful if the expert can provide peer-reviewed literature, or standards or instructional material published by national organizations such as NCCHC, APA, and ACA. Attorney Trey Yarbrough commented that: "The expert's depth of knowledge with respect to national and statewide standards and protocols relative to jail/prison management, supervision, and oversight" is a significant factor in choosing an expert besides his/her "history with other attorneys, the expert's perceived demeanor with respect to credibility, frankness, and transparency."

Being Authoritative and Relatable

Attorney Michael Zicolello emphasized that the bottom line is that the expert must be both authoritative and relatable because the ultimate test is whether the expert can convince a jury of twelve people with varying education and background that his or her opinions are the correct opinions, as opposed to those espoused by the opposing expert (because there is always an opposing expert).

Attorney Pari Scroggin stated that the expert witness must be able to tell the story in a relatable way to a jury and must present visually and audibly in a pleasing manner—not be hyper-technical in word choices, yet coming across as authoritative.

Attorney John Ray wrote: "The most important factor that I consider is their relatability to the jury. Therefore, I try to determine who I believe will be able to establish a connection with the jurors, based on his or her professional and personal connection to the local community, the depth of his or her experience and knowledge within that community, and his or her personality."

Persuasiveness and Communication

By and large, the jury will not have scientific, medical, or technical training. Therefore, experts must be able to make complex professional issues easily understandable in a relatively short amount of time. This does not mean that the expert necessarily must have previous testifying experience, though that is preferable.

The expert must communicate freely, even bluntly, and not be offended by aggressive challenges during consultation.

Attorney Eric Schoonveld stated, "Good experts are good educators. They need to be objective and not afraid to tell the attorney the bad news. Attorneys prefer an honest opinion on issues."

An expert can have outstanding knowledge in the field, but must effectively communicate his/her opinions clearly and concisely. Experts must relate to the common person and develop practical examples to explain complex subjects quickly, concisely, and accurately. In other words, the expert should effectively communicate his opinions so that an eighth grader can understand them. He/she must be able to relate to a jury and convey complexities straightforwardly and understandably.

Attorney Grabarek noted that: "An expert is effective if he has a sense as to how the jury perceives the expert. In my experience, jurors feel that an expert is effective when the expert limits the number of points he imparts to the jury. The expert should lay out his points during the initial phase of his testimony. This is akin to a road map. The expert can make it clear where he is going and how he will arrive there. The points that are imparted will, if presented correctly, remain in the minds of the jurors throughout the trial." If the expert is succinct, he will establish a great deal of credibility with the jury. He will also be more likely to have a favorable impact on the jury because the jurors are more likely to recall the points imparted by the clear and laconic expert.

Jurors become frustrated and irritated when they feel that their time is being wasted. Prospective jurors spend a significant amount of time waiting for the jury selection process to be completed. Furthermore, jurors are often sequestered, by necessity, during the inevitable last-minute pretrial hearings. Jurors are mindful when any witness or any lawyer drones on and on. Unfortunately, this is a common occurrence.

Exclusion of Opinions

Attorney Frederickson stated that litigants routinely ask courts to exclude their opponent's experts from testifying. There are a variety of reasons a court may do so. It does not, therefore, preclude an attorney from hiring an expert. But it is important to investigate why an expert may have been excluded from testifying in a prior case.

An attorney commented that Daubert motions are now overused. Some attorneys file Daubert motions against almost every expert. Another attorney commented that he is reluctant to file Daubert motions because he is concerned that he would be giving away his strategy to cross-examine the expert.

An attorney commented that he had success striking scientific experts on 702 factors 1, 3, and 4 (a reference to state court list noted, which are derived from the federal factors anyway). In a deposition, he would ask whether the expert has considered other explanations (other than the one in his opinion) and why he excludes them. He would further ask questions seeking to explain all systems he employed to determine the likelihood that his opinion is incorrect. He further commented, "These questions are not always appropriate for the reasons above— how would a jackhammer expert answer those questions, and why should he? But almost always, the answers to these lines of questions are unsatisfying, meaning the bad answers are useful to me when challenging the opinions/witnesses. On the other side of the coin, I prepare my own witnesses in advance to address these issues and avoid the disqualification traps."

Attorney Paul Messing wrote that: "An expert must demonstrate compliance with the Daubert standards: there must be a showing that the expert's theory can be (or has been) tested by experts in the field; that it has been subject to peer review; there should be an acknowledgment of the known or potential rate of error in the theory; and whether the theory is generally accepted in the relevant community. Separately, there must be a showing of the 'fit' that is required of any expert testimony, that it is relevant to the issues to be decided in the case. Finally, if an expert's testimony on issues of law is inadmissible, any opinion must not contain an impermissible legal conclusion which improperly intrudes upon the exclusive province of the court."

In many attorneys' experiences, most judges are reluctant to exclude experts.

Cost Considerations

For some attorneys, cost is of paramount importance. While expert costs are expensive, experts who charge outrageous amounts are not always favorably considered. However, if the expert is genuine, credible, and persuasive, expert fee is not a major consideration for the jury.

CONCLUSION

Most attorneys take their responsibility in hiring experts seriously. Individual attorneys choose experts by their personal and professional experience and requirements beyond what is required per Rule 702. The experts who are knowledgeable, genuine, credible, persuasive, and relatable contribute significantly to the outcome of a lawsuit. The jury, as the trier of fact, is the ultimate decision-maker of a case.

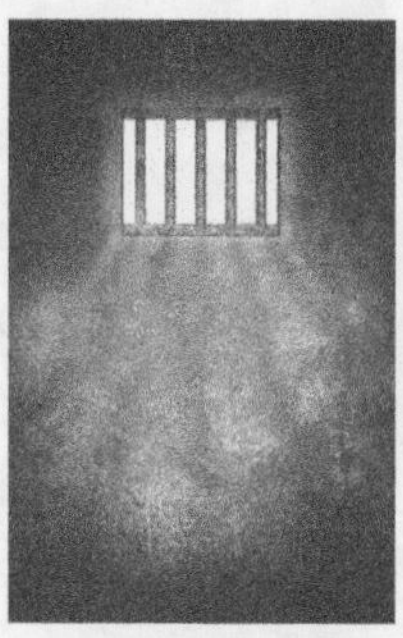

CONCLUSION

I wrote *Suicide in Jails and Prisons: Preventive and Legal Perspectives* with a firm conviction that most suicides in jails and prisons are preventable. To that end, I share my experience and expertise acquired over several decades in mental health and correctional psychiatry.

The goal of this book is twofold. First, it educates the readers about the who, how, and why of suicide in jails and prisons: who is at risk, what methods they use to make their attempts, and why they do it. It offers specific, actionable guidelines on how to avoid these suicides, including curricula for training correctional officials. Second, the book gives information and advice for the experts and legal professionals involved in the lawsuits that result from suicides.

Inmates are among the most vulnerable group for suicide. While many inmates decide to harm themselves impulsively, the telltale and predictable warning signs, if captured, provide an opportunity to save their lives. Suicidal thoughts and behaviors are transient, reflecting the paradox of the phenomenon of suicide in jails and prisons.

I emphasize that the best model for suicide prevention is the stakeholders' collective multidisciplinary approach. Each professional performs the assigned duty knowing full well his/her role, with a clear understanding of the requisite policies, procedures, and practice. Training, perhaps the most important component of suicide prevention, is crucial.

The best practices of mental health treatment of inmates reduce the instances of morbidity as well as mortality by suicide among this vulnerable population. Quality improvement of services is a desirable goal. Accordingly, clinical and programmatic information related to suicides and suicide attempts enable correctional officials to provide the best possible treatment for them. No matter our attitude toward inmates, we must provide the best professional judgment in monitoring, intervention, treatment, and supervision—despite their background and history.

A substantial number of suicides are followed by lawsuits. This is a significant issue that demands careful attention. The best practices in suicide prevention save lives and are a strong defense against legal action by the survivors. The book discusses the lessons learned over the past four decades in suicide-related litigation, especially from a historical perspective, and how court decisions have evolved. Yet there is a long way to go to set the guidance, standards, and parameters for court decisions, recognizing full well the subjective aspect of jury decisions.

Providing expert witness testimony is anxiety provoking even to the most experienced professionals. I offer specific guidance on how to perform the study and analysis of litigation claims of civil rights violations involving suicide or attempted suicide. In addition, valuable guidance to experts is offered, as well as how to be an effective witness in a court of law. The ultimate performance venue of an expert is the court of law.

The unique property of this book is the discussion of the legal aspects of inmate suicide in the context of preventive efforts. In this regard, the book will give attorneys a greater understanding of the issues involved in suicide prevention. The families of the deceased will also find this book informative.

Suicide in Jails and Prisons: Preventive and Legal Perspectives will be an invaluable resource for mental health professionals, correctional workers, attorneys, and even the families of incarcerated individuals who have died by suicide. It is a useful addition to the existing limited literature on prevention and litigation. The book paves the way for further research, studies, and shared knowledge.

—Anasseril E. Daniel, MD

SUICIDE PREVENTION TRAINING OUTLINE

By Anasseril E. Daniel, MD
and Lt. Richard Lichten (Ret.)

Training is the only tool that accomplishes the dual goal of preventing suicides and avoiding lawsuits. The World Health Organization (WHO) Resource Guide to Prevent Suicide In Jails and Prisons, An Update (2006) emphasizes that the essential component of any suicide prevention program is the properly trained correctional staff, who form the backbone of any jail, prison, and detention facility.

Each facility must identify the objectives of training that must include suicide awareness and identification of inmates at risk so the staff can take appropriate steps to monitor, intervene, and treat them.

INSTRUCTIONAL OBJECTIVES

The facility's training mission statement should establish that most, but not all, suicides are preventable. Based on the mission, the administration must create an attitude among the staff that knowledge and awareness of the training objectives of suicide prevention will save lives.

The objectives of the suicide prevention training should:

1. help the staff develop knowledge on factors that cause or contribute to the suicide risk of an inmate, with the understanding that jails and prisons are high-risk environments and situational stressors often act as a precipitant of suicide;
2. help staff screen, identify, and assess behavior signs and symptoms indicating potential suicide risk;
3. make the staff aware of mental and emotional signs and symptoms contributing to inmate suicidal behaviors;
4. educate the staff on techniques of intervention and monitoring of the inmate;
5. facilitate communication with the inmate during an actual suicide attempt and gesture;
6. train the staff on the facility's policy, procedures, and practice-related suicide screening, identification, assessment, intervention, and monitoring at-risk inmates;
7. train the staff on intervention procedures and protocols after a completed suicide, including proper documentation; and
8. train the correctional officers on general suicide prevention programs and strategies as well as on discipline-specific procedures and practice.

WHO SHOULD UNDERGO TRAINING?

All correctional, mental health, and medical staff must receive suicide prevention training. Newly assigned correctional officers should have suicide prevention training as soon as possible, preferably before the start of their first shift. Administrators, including the jail commander, should actively participate in the training sessions so that the correctional staff can become familiar with their expectations and concerns.

HOW OFTEN?

The standard training comprises four hours of didactic lectures at the time of employee hire and two hours of refresher course annually.

WHO PROVIDES THE TRAINING?

Most new employees receive their initial training at their state academy of training. The refresher course must be offered at the specific facilities by trained trainers. Videos of suicide vignettes depicting various scenarios of screening, assessment, post-suicide attempts, and post suicidal procedures will be helpful.

The training instructors must be well trained in preventing suicides and know the facility policies, procedures, and practices.

Contractors, if used by the facility, have the primary responsibility of training the assigned employees; however, they must do the training in collaboration with the contracting facility.

Most jails and prisons use licensed mental health professionals to perform suicide-risk assessment. An unlicensed professional, if assigned to perform suicide-risk assessment, requires intensive training. Besides didactic lectures and computer vignettes, a licensed mental health professional must provide direct hands-on supervision of the employee of at least five suicide risk assessments and post-assessment procedures. To avoid or to defend a liability claim, meticulous documentation of training must be kept on the employee's personnel file.

MODULE 1: MYTHS/FACTS OF SUICIDE

The training module must comprise an open discussion of myths and facts about suicide.

1. *Myth:* Suicides cannot be prevented.
    Fact: With proper procedure and practice, most suicides can be prevented.

2. *Myth:* Once an inmate decides on suicide, nothing can be done.
    Fact: Suicidal thoughts are transient. A candid discussion of the stressors often discourages the inmate from taking his/her life and allows the provider to help the inmate deal with the stress. Kindness and communication are the keys to avert suicide.

3. *Myth:* People who engage in suicidal gestures or threaten suicide are manipulative.
    Fact: While inmates may engage in suicidal gestures for attention seeking, death can occur during such gestures.

4. *Myth:* You should not ask about suicidal ideation, intent, and plan because it will give the inmate ideas.
    Fact: Asking about suicidal ideation will allow the inmates to vent their frustration and understand their feelings and thoughts. Furthermore, it is the standard of care.

5. *Myth:* Anyone who tries to kill themself is crazy.
   Fact: While most inmates who attempt suicide have a diagnosis of a mental disorder/s, they should not be considered crazy in the colloquial sense.

6. *Myth:* Genuinely suicidal inmates always admit to having suicidal thoughts.
   Fact: Most inmates with true intent conceal their ideation to avoid being placed in a suicide observation cell with almost no personal belongings.

7. *Myth:* Women do not commit suicide.
   Fact: Women attempt suicide more often than men, and mentally ill female inmates who attempt suicide die more often than men.

MODULE 2: STATISTICS AND RISK FACTORS

The training module must include a discussion of various terms related to suicide (Chapter 1), statistics of suicide in jails and prisons (Chapter 2), risk and protective factors (Chapter 3), and key facts as noted below:

1. Inmates are a high-risk group for suicide.
2. Suicide is the leading cause of death in jails and the third cause of death in prisons.
3. The incidence of suicide in jails and prisons is higher than in the general population.
4. Hanging is the predominant method of suicide.
5. Men commit suicide more often than women.
6. Past near-suicide attempt increases suicide vulnerability.

7. Depression, hopelessness, and anxiety are the predominant mental states among suicidal inmates.
8. Intoxication with alcohol and opiates is correlated with suicide in jails during the early period of detention.
9. Suicide and wrongful deaths are the leading causes of litigation related to jails and prisons.

MODULE 3: HIGH-RISK INMATE PROFILE AND SITUATIONAL FACTORS

1. Inmates with a past and current history of mental disorders, particularly with symptoms such as depression, anxiety, agitation, insomnia, and hopelessness
2. Verbal threats of suicide and current suicidal ideation
3. Recent history of near-lethal suicide attempt
4. First seven days of detention, particularly for those with alcohol or opiate intoxication at the time of detention
5. First-time detentions of those of high status in society
6. Loss of resources or support and rejection from family and friends
7. Unexpectedly long and harsh sentences and unfavorable court proceedings
8. A charge/s of heinous crime including rape and sexual assault of a minor
9. Placement in Maximum Security Unit or Administrative Segregation
10. Repeated placements on crisis watches
11. Inmates with withdrawal, isolation, giving away possessions, feeling sad, feeling worthless, and refusing treatment

MODULE 4: MENTAL DISORDERS

The following topics should be the focus of training, preferably provided by a psychologist or psychiatrist:

1. Signs and symptoms of mental disorder
2. Basics of diagnosis of mental disorders per DSM-5
   a. Depressive disorder
   b. Anxiety disorder
   c. Psychotic disorder
3. Verbal and behavior cues of mentally ill individuals
4. Impact of situational stressors on the mental state
5. Breakthrough symptoms of mental illness in otherwise stable mentally ill inmates
6. Substance abuse, intoxication, and withdrawal
7. Psychotropic medications and side effects
8. Referral of mentally ill inmates for treatment

MODULE 5: SCREENING, RISK ASSESSMENT, SUICIDE WATCH

1. Procedures of completing suicide screening (all staff)
2. Documentation of screening results (all staff)
3. Communication (all staff)
4. Risk Assessment (Mental Health Professionals)
5. Suicide watch logs and record-keeping
6. Review of records (jail and community sources)
7. Release of Information
8. Scheduling appointments
9. Processing and triaging of Medical Services Requests (MSR)
10. Administrative segregation rounds

MODULE 6: POLICIES, PROCEDURES, AND PRACTICE

1. Suicide prevention and intervention (all staff)
2. Access to mental health care (all staff)
3. Emergency management measures (all staff)
4. Psychotropic medication management (medical and mental health staff)
5. Involuntary medication administration (medical and mental health staff)
6. Transfer to an outside psychiatric facility (medical and mental health staff)

MODULE 7: CORRECTIONAL OFFICERS

The correctional officers should be aware of the medical staff and mental health staff's responsibilities and the policies and procedures related to suicide prevention.

The staff must regularly review the plan at shift briefing: roll call, etc. The training provided to the correctional officers must be ongoing, verifiable (well documented), and as realistic as possible. For example, role play a response to an inmate hanging attempt.

Training correctional officers must focus on several key areas of care and supervision:

1. Procedures to gather information from the arresting officers
2. Procedures to complete the screening questionnaire
3. Procedures to identify inmates at risk and post identification procedures, including placing inmates on suicide watch and monitoring

4. Documentation of observation and decisions after screening
5. Communication of potential suicide risk of an inmate to mental health professionals
6. Suicide watch and logs and inmate safety checks
7. Classification procedures and housing assignment
8. Incident report completion requirements and management
9. Emergency management procedures
10. Medication dispensation practices, if assigned
11. Use of restraints
12. The proper method of inspecting cells and dorms for likely ligature (noose) anchor points such as towel hooks that do not "break"
13. Inspection of the length of telephone cords on inmates' telephones
14. Inspection of the intercom system
15. Inspection of rescue tool or cut-down device in the case of hanging. The staff must be fully trained in using these cut-down tools and practice with them during rescue drills.
16. Training on de-escalation for the line staff.
17. Correctional officers may encounter an inmate in the process of suicide, and the staff should have the verbal tools to render the situation safe.
18. The Hospital Insurance Portability and Accountability Act (HIPAA) regulations

DETOXIFICATION PROTOCOLS

Fred Rottnek, MD

The ability of medical providers to detoxify effectively and safely—or detox—patients from alcohol or opioids is highly dependent on the resources in the facility.

All facilities that can monitor a detainee's orientation, respiratory rate, pulse, and blood pressure can offer comfort medications under a physician's standing order or protocol. If a facility has an infirmary or dedicated medical area, the facility can—in fact, should—offer comfort medications as well as other medications that promote safe and effective detox.

ALCOHOL DETOXIFICATION TEMPLATE

The guidelines noted are a starting point for physicians to create a protocol for alcohol detox. They are not intended to be definitive; rather, they are intended to be a starting point for physicians to adapt.

The medical director must assess the medical resources in the facility for medically monitored detox, (i.e., detox facilitated by use of medications, particularly use of benzodiazepines). Is there 24/7 staffing of registered nurses or other licensed professionals who can provide clinical assessments? Is there a 24/7 on-call medical prescribing provider coverage? Does the facility have the ability to monitor breath alcohol levels? And does the facility have adequate staffing to inventory and administer benzodiazepines if indicated for alcohol withdrawal detox?

Lack of any of the resources above is a useful prompt to send a detainee out to a local hospital or sobering center for medically monitored detox. More specific criteria for sending a detainee out for medically monitored detox include:

- Breath/Blood Alcohol Level (BAL) greater than 0.3 (measured in grams of ethanol, in 100 milliliters of blood, or 210 liters of breath)

- PAWSS Score (Prediction of Alcohol Withdrawal Severity Scale[2]) > 4

- Presence of co-occurring mental illness

- Concern for polysubstance use

---

2 Maldonado JR, Sher Y, Ashouri JF, Hills-Evans K, Swendsen H, Lolak S, Miller AC. The "Prediction of Alcohol Withdrawal Severity Scale" (PAWSS): Systematic literature review and pilot study of a new scale for the prediction of complicated alcohol withdrawal syndrome. Alcohol. 2014 Jun; 48(4):375–90. doi: 10.1016/j.alcohol.2014.01.004. Epub 2014 Feb 19. PMID: 24657098.

ALCOHOL DETOXIFICATION FOR CORRECTIONAL FACILITIES WITH 24/7 MEDICAL SERVICES

Conduct and document PAWSS. A score > 4 suggests that a patient is at risk for a more complicated withdrawal process. If an inmate scores 3 or less, consider housing in the general population with nursing assessments and medications every shift.

Process for patient detox in general population (PAWSS score of 3 or less with no co-occurring disorders)

1. Monitor patient orientation every shift and as needed to promote patient safety

2. Encourage hydration prior to and during the withdrawal process. Encourage a minimum of eight 8-oz glasses of water per day. Encourage sips, not gulping. Encourage use of ice chips, if available.

3. Encourage the patient to use comfort medications. Follow standard institutional processes for consent and patient education.

MEDICATIONS

   a. Trazodone 100 mg: Take one tablet daily 30 mins before bedtime as needed for sleep. Allow 7 to 8 hours of sleep (#10) (no routine refill) (Note: Educate patient that this is not an FDA-approved medication for insomnia; however, it is routinely used to alleviate this symptom during alcohol detox.)

   b. Compazine 10 mg: Take one tablet three times daily as needed for nausea (#30) (no routine refill)

   c. Clonidine 0.1 mg: Take one tablet every 12 hours daily as needed for anxiety, agitation, rapid heart rate, headache (#20) Hold for BP less than 100/60 (no routine refill) (Note: Educate patient that this is not an FDA-approved medication for alcohol detox; however, it is routinely used to alleviate this symptom during alcohol detox).

Detoxification in medical infirmary (if available, for PAWSS scores > 4 or if medical staff has additional concerns for complicated withdrawal)

1. IV Fluids
   a. Assess for contraindication or caution for IV fluid administration
   b. Baseline: 0.5 normal saline 200 cc/hour x 2 liters
   c. Continue if there are ongoing signs and symptoms of dehydration

2. Encourage hydration during the withdrawal process. Encourage a minimum of eight 8-oz glasses of water per day. Encourage sips, not gulping. Encourage use of ice chips, if available.

3. Medications—Benzodiazepine Protocol
   a. Chlordiazepoxide 25 mg (alternative, lorazepam 1 mg)
      i. Dosing schedule
         A. Take 1 capsule every 6 hours for the first 2 days

    B. Take 1 capsule every 8 hours for the next 2 days

    C. Take 1 capsule every 12 hours for the next 2 days

    D. Take 1 capsule every 24 hours for the final 2 days (no routine refill)

i. Patient should be drowsy but arousable

    A. If patient is not adequately sedated, consider doubling the dose for the first 2 to 4 days.

    B. If patient is not adequately sedated with the above increased benzodiazepine dose, consider adding haloperidol every 6 hours as needed to provide adequate sedation.

    i. Scheduled dosing with benzodiazepines is recommended over sign/symptom-driven dosing because most correctional facilities have minimal nurse staffing.[3]

    Scheduled dosing tends to be more effective for facilities with fewer nurses.

    ii. Consider benzodiazepine-sparing protocols for your institution.[4]

b. Folic Acid (Vitamin B9) 1 mg: Take 1 tablet daily for 14 days (no routine refill)

c. Thiamine (Vitamin B1) 100 mg: Take 1 tablet daily for 14 days (no routine refill)

---

3 Scheduled dosing of BZDs

4 See Maldonado JR. Novel Algorithms for the Prophylaxis and Management of Alcohol Withdrawal Syndromes-Beyond Benzodiazepines. Crit Care Clin. 2017 Jul;33(3):559–599. doi: 10.1016/j.ccc.2017.03.012. PMID: 28601135.

d. Seizure prophylaxis medications: Choose one if client has had history of complicated alcohol withdrawal

    A. Carbamazepine 200 orally two times daily for 7 days (Note: Educate patient that this is not an FDA-approved medication for seizure prophylaxis; however, it is routinely used to alleviate this symptom during alcohol detox.)

    B. Gabapentin 300 orally three times daily for 7 days (Note: Educate patient that this is not an FDA-approved medication for seizure prophylaxis; however, it is routinely used to alleviate this symptom during alcohol detox.)

4. Encourage the patient to use comfort medications. Follow standard institutional processes for consent and patient education.

MEDICATIONS

a. Trazodone 100 mg: Take one tablet daily 30 mins before bedtime as needed for sleep. Allow 7 to 8 hours of sleep (#10) (no routine refill) (Note: Educate patient that this is not an FDA-approved medication for insomnia; however, it is routinely used to alleviate this symptom during alcohol detox.)

b. Compazine 10 mg: Take one tablet three times daily as needed for nausea (#30) (no routine refill)

c. Clonidine 0.1 mg: Take one tablet every 12 hours daily as needed for anxiety, agitation, rapid heart rate, headache (#20) Hold for BP less than 100/60 (no routine refill) (Note: Educate patient that this is not an FDA-approved medication for alcohol detox; however, it is routinely used to alleviate this symptom during alcohol detox.)

LABS AND OTHER MONITORING:

1. Initial labs
   a. CMP, CBC
   b. Qualitative HCG (hold medications until results are obtained; adjust medications as needed for pregnancy)
   c. UDS (for identification of any other substances that may complicate the detox process)
2. Monitor per institutional protocol for detox

OPIOID DETOXIFICATION FOR CORRECTIONAL FACILITIES WITH 24/7 MEDICAL SERVICES
The ability of medical providers to effectively and safely detoxify (or detox) patients from opioids is highly dependent on the resources in the facility.

All facilities with the ability to monitor a detainee's orientation, respiratory rate, pulse, and blood pressure can offer comfort medications under a physician's standing order or protocol.

OPIOID DETOXIFICATION TEMPLATE
The guidelines noted are a starting point for physicians to cre-ate a protocol for alcohol detox. They are not intended to be

definitive; rather, they are intended to be a starting point for physicians to adapt.

Lack of any of the resources previously noted is a useful prompt to send a detainee out to a local hospital or sobering center for medically monitored detox. More specific criteria for sending a detainee out for medically monitored detox include:

- presence of co-occurring mental illness;

- concern for polysubstance use; and

- use of more than one naloxone administration prior to the detainee's arrival at the facility (or within the facility).

ASSESSMENT AND SCREENING

Facilities should have urine drug screens (UDSs) that test for drugs common to the region. Traditional 6- and 7-panel screens do not test for semi-synthetic opioids (e.g., hydrocodone and oxycodone) or synthetic opioids (e.g., methadone and fentanyl).

SPECIAL NOTE ABOUT SYNTHETIC OPIOIDS AND UNPREDICTABLE PURITY OF DRUG SUPPLY

Current U.S. street drug supplies have become increasingly unpredictable in the purity and potency. Moreover, many drugs have been intentionally or unintentionally contaminated by other drugs of the same class (fentanyl in heroin) and drugs of other classes (high-dose methamphetamine in heroin or fentanyl).[5] Because of this unpredictability, intoxication and detox processes are often unpredictable and complicated. For this reason, naloxone should be readily available throughout the facility, and all correctional and medical staff should be trained on indications and administration of naloxone.

OPIOID DETOXIFICATION MEDICATIONS

1. Encourage hydration during the withdrawal process. Encourage a minimum of eight 8-oz glasses of water per day. Encourage sips, not gulping. Encourage use of ice chips, if available.

2. Encourage the patient to use comfort medications.

    a. Trazodone 100 mg: Take one tablet daily 30 mins before bedtime as needed for sleep. Allow 7 to 8 hours of sleep (#10) (no routine refill)

    b. Compazine 10 mg: Take one tablet three times daily as needed for nausea (#30) (no routine refill)

    c. Clonidine 0.1 mg: Take one tablet every 12 hours daily as needed for anxiety, agitation, rapid heart rate, headache (#20) Hold for BP less than 100/60 (no routine refill)

    d. Baclofen 10 mg orally three times daily as needed for cramping (#30) (no routine refill) or Flexeril 10 mg: Take one tablet every 8 hours as needed for muscle cramping (#30) (no routine refill)

---

5 FACING ADDICTION IN AMERICA The Surgeon General's Spotlight on Opioids, https://addiction.surgeongeneral.gov/sites/default/files/Spotlight-on-Opioids_09192018.pdf

LABS AND OTHER MONITORING:

1. Initial labs
   a. CMP, CBC
   b. Qualitative HCG (hold medications until results are obtained; adjust medications as needed for pregnancy)
   c. UDS (for identification of any other substances that may complicate the detox process)
2. Monitor per institutional protocol for detox

PROVIDING MEDICATIONS FOR ALCOHOL AND OPIOID USE DISORDER TREATMENT AND RELAPSE PREVENTION, OR WHAT HAPPENS AFTER DETOX?

Professional organizations are nearly unanimous in their advocacy for initiation of opioid use disorder treatment for detainees while in custody. These organizations include the National Sheriffs' Association,[6] the National Commission for Correctional Health Care,[7] the Substance Abuse and Mental Health Services Administration,[8] and the Prison Policy Initiative.[9]

---

6 Jail-Based Medication-Assisted Treatment Promising Practices, Guidelines, and Resources for the Field https://www.sheriffs.org/publications/Jail-Based -MAT-PPG.pdf

7 Jail-Based MAT: Promising Practices, Guidelines and Resources https:// www.ncchc.org/jail-based-MAT

8 Medication-Assisted Treatment (MAT) in the Criminal Justice System: Brief Guidance to States, https://store.samhsa.gov/sites/default/files/d7/priv /pep19-matbriefcjs_0.pdf

9 We know how to prevent opioid overdose deaths for people leaving prison. So why are prisons doing nothing? https://www.prisonpolicy.org /blog/2018/12/07/opioids/

However, many facilities do not have the medical staff to evaluate, treat, and start or maintain patients on medications for substance-use disorders (SUDs). The following are medication recommendations that can be done with a commitment to the work.

JAILS

Jail stays are often unpredictable, and release of inmates is often unannounced. However, some jails, including the Saint Louis County (Missouri) Jail and jails in Rhode Island,[10] have been able to maintain patients on medications that nursing staff confirm in the jail community.

A challenge for patients and providers in a jail is determining the best course of treatment for an individual whose legal problems are not settled, and the patient remains in custody but is being transferred to another facility. When a patient is being transferred to another facility, the provider should work with correctional staff and mental health staff to determine if SUD medication is available at the next facility. If SUD medication is provided, the patient's treatment can

---

10 This State Has Figured Out How to Treat Drug-Addicted Inmates https://www.pewtrusts.org/en/research-and-analysis/blogs/stateline/2020/02/26/this-state-has-figured-out-how-to-treat-drug-addicted-inmates

- Buprenorphine doses are continued at documented doses. Patients in the drug treatment program can initiate buprenorphine treatment as well.
- Patients on extended-release naltrexone (for alcohol and/or opioid use disorder) are maintained on daily oral naltrexone until their legal situation is resolved. If these patients are released back to community, they receive a depot formulation of extended-release naltrexone prior to discharge.
- Patients on methadone are continued on daily methadone treatment. The facility has arranged treatment with a local opioid treatment program so that patients have an evaluation every 14 days. The jail medical staff receive a 14-day supply for any patient on methadone.

continue uninterrupted. However, if the next facility does not provide SUD medications, the provider should discuss with the patient when the patient prefers to taper medications in the current medication program or face an abrupt discontinuation of medications at the next facility. A somewhat rapid taper at the current facility, with the comfort medications provided above, is usually the more comfortable option. If this is the treatment plan, the provider should prescribe comfort medications, as outlined above, with a taper such as the following:

Stabilization Dose	8 mg	16 mg	24 mg
Day 1	8	16	24
Day 2	6	12	20
Day 3	6	10	16
Day 4	4	8	12
Day 5	4	4	8
Day 6	2	2	4
Day 7	2	2	2

PRISONS

Most prisons do not routinely offer medications for SUDs. However, more prisons have begun treating patients with medications for SUDs, and this trend will likely expand. Massachusetts and Rhode Island have documented outcomes.

Discharges from prisons are more predictable. This predictability allows time for bridge programming with SUD providers in an individual's home plan. It also allows for initiation of any of the medications previously mentioned.

REFERENCES

References that supports the use of clonidine in opioid detoxification

1. Agren H. Clonidine treatment of the opiate withdrawal syndrome. A review of clinical trials of a theory. Acta Psychiatr Scand Suppl. 1986;327:91-113. PMID: 3529831.

2. Kleber HD, Gold MS, Riordan CE. The use of clonidine in detoxification from opiates. Bull Narc. 1980;32(2): 1-10. PMID: 6907020.

3. Kleber HD. Pharmacologic treatments for opioid dependence: detoxification and maintenance options. Dialogues Clin Neurosci. 2007;9(4):455-470. doi:10.31887 /DCNS.2007.9.2/hkleber

4. Up to Date, Medically supervised opioid withdrawal during treatment for addiction, https://www.uptodate. com/contents/medically-supervised-opioid-withdrawal -during-treatment-for-addiction

CHECKLIST FOR SUICIDE PREVENTION

ADMINISTRATORS: A FIFTEEN-POINT CHECKLIST

1. Establish an adequate mental health services delivery system.
2. Ensure compliance with applicable laws, state statutes, and administrative codes in setting policies and procedures, employee hiring and staffing.
3. Secure accreditations from National Commission of Correctional Healthcare (NCCHC), if possible.
4. Ensure and monitor contract compliance by private vendors of mental health services, medical services, and pharmacy.
5. Organize and administer suicide-prevention training and periodic refresher courses for all administrative, clinical, and custody/jail staff.
6. Establish a mechanism and procedure to consider suicide risk in offender housing, cell placement, and work assignments.

7. Ensure prompt transfer of mental health records of high-risk inmates from facility to facility and arrange for detailed information from jails transfer to prisons.

8. Develop procedures for handling inmate verbal and nonverbal communications of intent to harm self.

9. Ensure 24-hour access to emergency medical and mental health care.

10. Place inmates on suicide watch in line of sight or special observation cell.

11. Maintain suicide watch log consistent with policy.

12. Institute procedures for written clearance from mental health staff before transferring an offender on suicide watch to the general population or to other cells.

13. Set up a mechanism to receive, document, and transmit to mental health staff information from family.

14. Set up periodic audits of health care and mental health care policies and procedures.

15. Appoint a suicide prevention coordinator.

PSYCHOLOGISTS, SOCIAL WORKERS, MENTAL HEALTH PROFESSIONALS, THERAPISTS: FIFTEEN-POINT CHECKLIST

1. Perform routine and thorough intake screenings.

2. Perform detailed suicide screenings.

3. Develop an initial treatment plan using the data from screening procedures.

4. Gather inmate mental health history from community sources.

5. Perform a mental health evaluation when inmates screen positive and modify the treatment plan based on findings.

6. Determine the need for placement of inmates on suicide watch.

7. Provide input to correctional staff for cell assignment and housing.

8. Conduct suicide-risk assessments regularly and when indicated—including at every health-care encounter.

9. Perform suicide risk assessments when inmates return from out-count.

10. Perform suicide risk assessment after court appearances, a new sentence, or any major psychosocial stressor.

11. Specify suicide-watch procedures and communicate to administration and/or custody staff.

12. Monitor all high-risk inmates and those on suicide watch daily, consistent with the suicide prevention policy of the institution and professional standards.

13. Conduct weekly clinical and administrative rounds of inmates in solitary confinement; document mental status changes.

14. Treat at-risk individuals with appropriate clinical interventions including crisis intervention and supportive therapy.

15. Document all assessments, decisions, and actions.

PSYCHIATRISTS: FIFTEEN-POINT CHECKLIST

1. Conduct psychiatric evaluation to include a detailed mental status examination and DSM-5 diagnosis consistent with professional standards and guidelines.

2. Review clinician's notes and incident reports before a psychiatric visit.

3. Perform suicide risk assessment.
4. Develop a treatment plan when indicated.
5. initiate medication management if indicated.
6. Place inmates on substance withdrawal protocol if indicated.
7. Avoid abrupt discontinuation of medications of incoming inmate.
8. Provide bridge medications for those who are admitted to a jail and when transferred from jail to prison or prison to prison.
9. Conduct follow up visits and lab workups as clinically indicated, consistent with standard of care and facility policy.
10. Complete Abnormal Involuntary Movements Scale when indicated.
11. Facilitate timely admission/commitment to inpatient units for those at imminent risk of suicide.
12. Initiate involuntary medication if indicated.
13. Minimize or avoid the use of psychotropic medications with lethal potential, especially Tricyclic antidepressants.
14. Monitor medication non-compliant inmates.
15. Document all assessments, decisions, and actions.

NURSES (REGISTERED NURSE, LICENSED PRACTICAL NURSE): ELEVEN-POINT CHECKLIST

1. Have inmates sign a release of information and get medical records from community source.
2. Verify medications with outside provider and pharmacy.

3. Gather information regarding diagnosis and the medication dose, form, and method of administration.
4. Obtain orders from physicians and document them.
5. Create Medication Administration Record—paper or electronic—and maintain documents of all medication administered.
6. Dispense psychotropic medication on watch-take basis and perform mouth checks for all inmates.
7. Assess inmates for any side effects of medications.
8. Triage Medical Services Requests per frequency indicated by institutional policy.
9. Schedule inmates for a psychiatric appointment in a timely manner, if the task is assigned to nursing.
10. Escalate clinical concerns to supervisor and/or provider as per clinical training and as indicated by institutional policy.
11. Perform emergency lifesaving measures when indicated.

CORRECTIONAL OFFICERS: TEN-POINT CHECKLIST

1. Monitor inmates for indications of suicide risk.
2. Report behavioral changes and inmate communications of suicidal intent to supervisors and appropriate clinical personnel.
3. Recognize suicide risk among all inmates, regardless of any inmate's history of manipulation and attention seeking.
4. Facilitate medical and mental health evaluations.
5. Conduct and document suicide watch accurately.
6. Perform safety checks in a timely manner and consistent with institutional policy.

7. Avoid intimidation and sexual coercion.
8. Perform thorough and individual suicide screening, if assigned.
9. Perform medication dispensation on a watch-take, including mouth checks, if assigned.
10. Perform lifesaving measures promptly.

APPENDIX 4

ATTORNEYS' PERSPECTIVES ON EXPERTS

1. MICHAEL ZICOLELLO, WILLIAMSPORT, PENNSYLVANIA

The factors I weigh are the extent of the expert's work experience in or with the prison system: Has the expert published any professional works on prison conditions and/or suicide; has the expert been a professor, lecturer, or spoken at seminars related to issues involving prison conditions and/or suicide; whether I feel I have a good rapport with the expert; and previous experience as a litigation expert in prison suicide cases.

I do not give any special weight to the factors set forth in Rule 702 other than ensuring that the expert will meet the requirements to provide expert testimony in federal court under the Daubert standard. The bottom line is that the expert must be both authoritative and relatable because the ultimate test is whether the expert can convince a jury of twelve people with varying educations and backgrounds that his opinions are the correct opinions, as opposed to those espoused by the opposing expert (because there is always an opposing expert).

—Michael J. Zicolello, Esq.
   SCHEMERY ZICOLELLO, P.C. 333 Market Street,
      Williamsport, PA 17701

2. PARI SCROGGIN, CHANDLER, ARIZONA

Federal Rules of Evidence 702 states that expert opinions are admissible if the expert's scientific, technical, or other specialized knowledge will help the trier of fact to understand the evidence or to determine a fact at issue, but to me, that very often is an easy hurdle to meet given the background knowledge of experts. Therefore, I select an expert with a jury trial in mind.

Like any witness in a case, experts are a way to present the defense story to a jury. The most important factor for me is how the jury will perceive the witness (likable, credible?) The expert witness must be able to tell the story in a relatable way to a jury and must present visually and audibly in a pleasing manner—so not hyper-technical in word choices, yet still coming across as authoritative. Visually—the witness must present professionally (not sloppy or "overpriced," like a hired gun). My best approach to selecting experts is through word-of-mouth references to get a historical perspective of how the expert presents to a jury.

—Pari K. Scroggin
   Grasso Law Firm, 2250 East Germann Road, Suite 10,
      Chandler, AZ 85286

3. KATHLEEN GRIFFITH, DETROIT, MICHIGAN

Aside from experts' experience in the field, I consider their knowledgeability and familiarity with the law. Most jail suicide cases involve §1983 civil rights claims, which can be complex and convoluted. Another factor is the expert's ability to handle difficult questions during a deposition. If an expert has difficulty explaining or supporting their findings in a deposition, chances are they will not present well as a witness during a trial. The deposition of an expert can make or break a case in terms of settlement negotiations before trial.

—Kathleen M. Griffith

Attorney, Garan Lucow Miller, P.C., 1155 Brewery Park Blvd., Ste. 200 | Detroit, MI 48207

4. AMANDA L. BRIDSON, DALLAS, TEXAS

In selecting an expert, our primary focus is whether the expert has sufficient and particularized education, training, or experience that closely aligns with the issues in our case.

When we seek an expert for our prison suicide case, we are drawn to an expert with a particularized area of expertise—mental health in the prison system. We do not think it would be sufficient to simply hire a psychiatrist to opine on the deceased's mental health conditions while she was incarcerated. We also feel that it would be insufficient to hire an expert on general prison protocols. Instead, we want an expert who can help the jury understand the unique demands that incarceration can have on a person's mental health and how prison can and should respond to a prisoner experiencing a mental health crisis. Expert's resume should demonstrate superior knowledge in both medicine and prison policy. The expert must be able to opine on all facets of a prison suicide claim—medical diagnosis and treatment, adequate suicide prevention policy, and whether an entity has acted in accordance with those policies.

We weigh the evidence of an expert's participation in other court cases and how judges have ruled on challenges to qualifications and opinions. Because other courts had found your opinions to be based on sound methods and reasoning, we felt good about our ability to withstand future Daubert challenges.

—*Amanda L. Bridson*
  Sumner Schick LLP, 3006 Cole Avenue, Dallas, TX 75204

5. ROBIN FRAZER CLARK, ATLANTA, GEORGIA

The most important factor is the amount of actual hands-on experience an expert has in the subject field. A person can also be an expert if she/he teaches the subject, but nothing surpasses actual experience. In a prison suicide case setting, if there is a claim for psychiatric malpractice for failure to treat an inmate appropriately with mental health care, I am looking for a psychiatrist who not only has the medical credentials, but who has also worked in or supervised medical or nursing staff in a correctional setting. Often, defendants argue in these prison cases that a different standard of care, (i.e., a lesser standard of care), applies in a correctional setting. This is not true, but you need an expert who has practiced or supervised staff in a correctional setting to be able to refute that argument through an Affidavit or deposition testimony. A psychiatrist in a normal office setting is technically qualified to do that. Still, they often have not supervised nursing staff in a correctional setting, so you must be careful to make sure a psychiatrist you are hiring to testify in this kind of case has that experience.

In Georgia and other states, we have a statute that the expert witness must have practiced in essentially that same type of medical practice as the defendant in the three of the last five years before the incident at issue or has taught or is teaching in that area of medical practice. Many physicians have retired, thinking they will have a second career as an expert witness in medical malpractice cases. That is not possible in Georgia. A retired physician who is not teaching would not qualify to testify. Although our expert witness statute is not a "same specialty" requirement, our appellate courts have interpreted the statute essentially to require that. If you don't have an expert in the same specialty, you do so at your own risk.

Other factors I consider include: Has the expert published in this area? Given lectures or taught at conferences and testified in other similar cases? Are there any appellate opinions in the U.S. that mention the expert and have concluded he or she is qualified in a similar case? Do you have copies of Daubert Motions and Orders on your expert? Has the expert trained correctional officers? Or nursing or medical staff in a prison setting? If the expert has done this training in what is known as a mental health prison, that is even better. Do others in the correctional field also consider him or her an expert in the field? Will a jury like him or her? Is the expert confident? Do they make a good impression?

Suppose there is a U.S. appellate opinion in which an appellate court has found that the expert is qualified as a matter of law. In that case, you will want to make sure you have that opinion as often; many courts need only for another court already to have ruled on the expert's qualifications in a particular field for the current court to bless the expert. You will also want to obtain as many Orders denying Daubert motions on the expert by trial judges as possible. What other trial judges have done on Daubert's motions on this expert is very persuasive to most sitting trial judges. It not only makes their job easier but also gives them confidence in ruling the expert may testify.

So, of those factors listed in Rule 702, I would say the most important one is qualifications, or as the statute says, "(a) knowledge, skill, experience, training or education . . ."

Counsel can handle the other three factors together with the expert if the expert is qualified.

A witness who is qualified as an expert by knowledge, skill, experience, training, or education may testify in the form of an opinion or otherwise if:

(a) the expert's scientific, technical, or other specialized knowledge will help the trier of fact understand the evidence or determine a fact in issue;

(b) the testimony is based on sufficient facts or data;

(c) the testimony is the product of reliable principles and methods; and

(d) the expert has reliably applied the principles and methods to the facts of the case. Fed. R. Evid. 702

—*Robin Frazer Clark*

  Fiftieth President of the State Bar of Georgia (2012–13),
  101 Marietta Street, N.W. Centennial Tower, Suite
  2300, Atlanta, GA 30303

6. ERIC FREDERICKSON, ATLANTA, GEORGIA

If the expert has the prerequisite qualifications to offer opinions in the area I need, the most important factor I consider is the expert's communications skills. The jury will not have medical training. Experts must be able to make complex medical issues easily understandable in a relatively short amount of time. This does not mean that the expert necessarily must have previous testifying experience, though that is preferable.

The second most important factor is the expert's particular clinical experience. The more experience the expert has working in similar situations to that involved in my case, the better. At the least, the expert must have experience treating patients with similar mental health needs to that of the suicide victim in my case. It is highly preferable, though not required, that the expert have experience working in a correctional facility or otherwise treating incarcerated patients.

A third factor is whether a court has ever excluded the expert from testifying in a case. Litigants routinely ask courts to exclude their opponent's experts from testifying, and there are various reasons a court may do so. It does not, therefore, preclude me from hiring an expert. But it is important to investigate why they may have been excluded from testifying in a prior case.

2. Are any or all factors noted in Rule 702 or any other factors given special weight?

Rule 702 provides:

A witness who is qualified as an expert by knowledge, skill, experience, training, or education may testify in the form of an opinion or otherwise if:

(a) the expert's scientific, technical, or other specialized knowledge will help the trier of fact understand the evidence or determine a fact in issue;

(b) the testimony is based on sufficient facts or data;

(c) the testimony is the product of reliable principles and methods; and

(d) the expert has reliably applied the principles and methods to the facts of the case.

When a medical doctor is offering opinions in an area in which they are Board Certified (i.e., psychiatry), there is rarely serious argument about whether they have "scientific, technical, or other specialized knowledge will help the trier of fact." As a practical matter, therefore, subparts (b) through (d) typically carry more weight in a court's analysis of expert opinions in medical fields.

To ensure that the "testimony is based on sufficient facts or data," it is important that experts be prepared to point to the specific evidence in the case (medical records, fact witness testimony, etc.) on which their opinions are based. Regarding "reliable principles and methods," experts should be able to show that the way they have analyzed the case is in line with methods generally used in their field. It is helpful if the expert can provide peer-reviewed literature, or standards, or instructional material published by authoritative bodies (i.e., the American College of Psychiatrists) that support their approach.

—Eric S. Fredrickson
Harman Law Firm LLC, 3575 Piedmont Rd Bldg. 15, Suite 1040, Atlanta, GA 30305

7. MARLON PRIMES, U.S. DISTRICT ATTORNEY, NORTHERN DISTRICT OF OHIO, CLEVELAND, OHIO

The key factors I examine in selecting an expert witness are as follows:

1. Knowledge in the relevant field. The expert's resume and background should indicate that he or she has an excellent understanding and mastery of their field of study. Consequently, I examine work and educational history that supports the notion that the expert really understands the subject matter, has participated in continuing education to ensure their knowledge is up to date, and has a history of being an expert in the area.

2. Are the expert's opinions in the mainstream and accepted by their peers? The expert needs to be respected in their field of study. Therefore, I closely examine memberships in professional organizations and specifically seek to determine if the expert has been asked to speak or write for recognized professional organizations and for recognized peer-reviewed journals and publications.

3. Communication skills. An expert can have outstanding knowledge in the field, but he must effectively communicate his opinions clearly and concisely. Therefore, I try to hire experts who can relate to the common person and develop practical examples to explain complex subjects quickly, concisely, and accurately. In other words, the expert should be able to effectively communicate his or her expert opinions so that a sixth grader can understand them.

4. Bias. I do not ever want to be associated with an expert that can be perceived as a hired gun. So, an expert that has experience testifying for plaintiffs and defendants is very valuable. In litigation, there are often competing experts, and you want the finder of fact to give your expert the benefit of the doubt because of their reputation for being even-handed and practical. If the expert has set guidelines for formulating his or her opinions, they should be applied equally to plaintiffs and defendants.

5. Prior expert testimony. I closely examine the prior expert testimony of the proposed expert witness. One of the key factors is whether the testimony of the expert has been previously excluded. Also, I look to see if the expert's prior testimony has been criticized by his or her peers. Many professional associations have detailed rules for testifying as an expert witness. The rules typically require the expert to testify accurately, honestly, and within his or her field of expertise. If the expert has been sanctioned for failing to do so, that is a big red flag for me.

6. Affiliation with a university or a professional practice. I try to make sure that my experts do not simply spend all or most of their time testifying as expert witnesses because this gives the impression that they are hired. I like to hire experts that teach at a university because it gives the impression that they are keeping up with the latest research in the field, as most universities have publication requirements for faculty. It is also important that the expert have a professional practice. This helps ensure that they have a practical, and not just an ivory-tower, view of the field.

—Marlon A. Primes
Assistant U.S. Attorney, Northern District of Ohio, 801 West Superior Avenue, Suite 400, Cleveland, OH 44113

8. ANITA KORWIN, ATLANTA, GEORGIA

The physician expert witness procurement process involves various factors, largely dependent on the nature of the case. For instance, if the matter involves a suicide in a jail or prison, then a physician practicing in psychiatric medicine is needed. A forensic psychiatrist or a psychiatrist with experience in the correctional setting is most appropriate in this situation.

Federal Rules of Evidence, 702, states that expert opinions are admissible if the expert's scientific, technical, or other specialized knowledge will help the trier of fact to understand the evidence or to determine a fact at issue.

When reviewing a case pertaining to the suicide of an incarcerated individual, it is important that the expert understands the unique challenges that can be encountered in the correctional setting. Therefore, having an expert with experience in areas such as correctional psychiatry, addiction medicine, and crisis intervention can be very valuable in assessing the medical facts as they relate to a legal matter.

I typically search for academic physicians and physicians that are published in the subject matter for which they will be opining. Also, I find it helpful to have a physician with a current board certification as well as fellowship training in the area in which they will render an opinion.

Another important consideration is to select an expert who was practicing during the time at which the incident occurred, so that their clinical knowledge base is relevant to that time frame.

After a physician is located, their Curriculum Vitae and fee schedule are requested. At this initial stage, it is important to note any state-specific requirements that may have been adopted for expert witness testimony. Some states have specific rules governing a testifying expert, so it is important to ensure that the expert meets these requirements before proceeding.

Once it has been confirmed that the expert is a good fit for the case thus far, then the vetting process begins. It is important to cover background information to determine if the physician has any type of legal or criminal history, whether personal or professional.

The testimony history of the potential expert is also pertinent to determine if they are experienced with legal matters. It is always helpful to have an expert with some testifying experience; however, the main goal is to find an expert that is well-versed with the clinical aspects.

Suicide in the correctional setting requires an expert who must be skilled at objectively evaluating psychiatric issues as they interconnect with the legal system. Beyond these fundamental attributes, the expert must also be able to effectively communicate their clinical opinions as they relate to the legal questions. Ultimately, the expert has a duty to educate and assist the trier of fact.

—Anita Korwin, BSN, RN, LNC, Korwin Consulting, P.O. Box 19086, Atlanta, GA 31126

9. PATRICK PROVENZALE, LISLE, ILLINOIS

What are the factors you weigh in choosing an expert to work on your case?

I will confess, before you asked me the question, I never gave the issue of expert selection much thought from an epistemic approach. Thinking about it critically, I understand selection of an expert witness to be a case-specific, and sometimes a rather ad hoc, endeavor. Reflecting on this, I imagine this is because, for my practice, so many variables come into play because I handle a wide gamut of cases—constitutional claims I handle brought under §1983 touch upon myriad areas of expertise, from police practices to institutional medical care to forensic sciences to sociology; medical malpractice cases I handle run the spectrum of medical specialties; insurance subrogation cases I handle involve civil engineering issues; and damages issues in Plaintiff's cases in general can call for opinions across varying disciplines, from economics to neuropsychology. Some areas of expertise have go-to experts generally recognized in the field as the authority, whereas other areas are so well understood and studied those experts are essentially interchangeable.

The selection process, despite how daunting it can be, is nonetheless crucial. Selection of an expert witness in a case in which the attorney feels expert testimony will be of benefit can be the most important decision an attorney makes in a case. So how do I approach such a crucial process when, in most cases, I know far too little about the actual expert discipline implicated, but still need to select an expert whose job is to be the best person to convince twelve people of the point I am trying to get across? In other words, what kind of person convinces people to listen to him or her, instead of the expert the other side will proffer?

Unless the selecting attorney has prior experience with the expert or has a solid referral from a familiar colleague vouching for the expert, answering this question, of course, becomes educated guesswork. In the absence of prior experience or a vouching, selection of an expert among the many, many professionals in any given field who may technically qualify as an "expert" is, frankly, fraught with risks. Will I waste the client's money? Will the expert be able to provide the opinions I need, or as importantly, will he or she be candid and tell me he can't give those opinions because they are too easily attacked on cross, or worse, risk being barred (and hopefully the candid moment comes sooner than later)?

To mitigate these risks and ensure that I select an expert who will give me not only candid opinions, good or bad, but also ample ammunition to argue to a jury to believe my expert, I try to focus my selection process using the following general factors, in order of their importance: (1) Qualifications (2) Personable Affect and (3) Cost.

Before I discuss navigation of these factors, there is a step I always do first, which is to try to educate myself as best I can on the subject matter of expertise. This accomplishes two things. First, I will hopefully find the names of experts who have prominently studied, taught, or published on the topic I am dealing with. This by itself is a good way to identify a potential expert. Second, when I do eventually communicate with whomever I reach out to, I won't sound like a dithering idiot. The best experts are highly selective themselves with the attorneys they choose to work with—a lawyer will do herself no favor if she contacts an expert and does not exhibit an acceptable level of understanding of the subject matter to have a meaningful preliminary discussion with the expert.

Having done my homework on the subject, then, here are the factors I consider, in their general order of importance to me:

1. Qualifications:
    Diversity of professional credentials
    Academic
    Practical
    Research
    Authorship / Peer-Reviewed
    Diversity of Expert Witness Experience
    Retained by both plaintiff and defendant
    Appointed by a Court a plus
    Qualified by a Court of law to testify
    Daubert or otherwise
    Ratio of consulting work vis-à-vis other professional
       work
    Significant imbalance is bad

2. Personable affect
   Must be able to relate to a jury and convey complexities
   in a straightforward and understandable manner
3. Cost/Focus
   Cost-conscious
   Open to instruction from counsel and relies on counsel
   to orient/focus facts to expert issues in the case

By far the most important factor is the expert's overall qualifications. To me, there are two parts to an expert's qualifications: issue expertise and experienced expertise. The subject matter of expertise will certainly drive the selection somewhat, but I prefer an expert who has specific expertise in the issue in question—if he has taught, written, or studied the specific issue in question, that is a plus.

In my opinion, it is a superior position to be able to tell a jury that my expert is the one other experts rely on for teaching, reference authority, or cutting-edge studies in the field. A helpful qualification is an expert who has been appointed by a state or federal court. This is rare but can be a significant fact to point out to a jury. Not as helpful, but certainly important, is an expert who has testified at trial in a federal court—this allows the attorney to highlight to the jury that the witness has been recognized by other federal court judges as an expert in the field.

Second in importance in my mind is showing independence. When it comes to expert witnesses, no expert will convince anyone of anything if there is suspicion of bias. It is the death knell for the expert. Everything an attorney can point out to demonstrate the expert's independence in the field will help her defend against an argument that the expert is just a hired gun, or worse, an issue advocate.

Third in importance is the expert's personality. This is a very subjective factor, but I generally like to small talk expert witnesses for a time during initial conversations to evaluate the personability and likeability factor of the witness. At the end of the day, it helps to believe someone if you like them.

Finally, I am always mindful of cost, but generally, I am a firm believer that you get what you pay for and expect the best witnesses to be expensive.

Are any or all factors noted in Rule 702 or any other factors given special weight?

There is no simple answer to this question. If I were to give a simple answer, it would be no, there is no one factor that is more important than others. They are all important because infirmity in any one area can result in the expert's opinions being barred from trial. Assuming the selection of the expert followed the above factors (so that qualifications is not an issue), if one factor is more likely to get an expert barred than any other, in my opinion, it is methodology (so basically, FRE402(c) and (d)). Under Daubert, the expert generally has to employ the same methodology she employs when practicing in the field of expertise.

Some experts do not employ their normal methodologies because the methodology does not really translate into litigation. For example, disciplines that require data collection or statistical sampling are easily barred if the expert's methodology is not baked into the discovery strategy. Early consultation with the expert about discovery issues may, therefore, be instrumental to the admissibility of her opinions later, but again, this entirely depends on numerous case-specific factors that are too variable to dissect.

—Patrick L. Provenzale
Ekl, Williams & Provenzale LLC, Two Arboretum Lakes, 901 Warrenville Road, Suite 175, Lisle, IL 60532

10. ERIC SCHOONVELD, CHICAGO, ILLINOIS

I look at several factors in choosing an expert. First, they need to have significant experience and knowledge on the issue in the case. I will often choose real-world experience more than academic credentials. Second, they need to be a good communicator/educator and able to clearly communicate their opinions. Experts with teaching expertise are often strong communicators. Good experts are true educators. Third, they need to be interested and responsive to the needs of the case. The best expert in the world who is too busy or not responsive can create more problems than solutions. Fourth, they need to be objective and not afraid to tell me bad news. I much prefer an honest opinion than someone who tells me that everything is great and ends up backtracking down the road.

Rule 702 is broad and an expert with significant experience in the given issue will nearly always comply with Rule 702. Once an expert meets a basic threshold of scientific, technical, or specialized knowledge, I look closely at the other factors mentioned above.

—Eric Schoonveld
Hall, Prangle, Schoonveld, 200 South Wacker Drive, Suite 3300, Chicago, IL 60606

10. AMY BORING, ESQUIRE, WILLIAMSPORT, PENNSYLVANIA

The Rules of Evidence provide a basis for admissibility when choosing an expert. Beyond that, there are a variety of factors that we consider when choosing an expert consultant or witness. The specific facts and needs of the case are going to determine whether any factor is given special weight. First, I take a good look at the case's specific facts and determine what it really is that I need the expert to discuss or clarify. Some of the things I look for include area of expertise, length of practice in the area, publications, experience in litigation, and current employment. These factors help narrow the field of potential experts. After speaking with a potential expert, I'm now looking at factors such as relatability, ease of conversation about the specific issues the case raises, and an evaluation of how the person reacts to the issue (such as a sense of passion about it). Overall, I want to utilize an expert that I feel is compatible with me because we are going to work together to effectively present the information to the judge or jury.

—Amy R. Boring, Esquire
Schemery Zicolello, P.C., 333 Market Street,
Williamsport, PA 17701

12. PAUL MESSING, PHILADELPHIA, PENNSYLVANIA

The parties in jail suicide litigation rely on expert consultants and witnesses to determine whether they have grounds to pursue a case and, if so, whether they can prove or rebut liability. It is virtually impossible for a plaintiff to demonstrate liability without expert support.

Under the standards set forth in *Kumho Tire* and Daubert, Rule 702 permits the introduction of expert testimony only where the proponent establishes by a preponderance of the evidence that the proposed expert is qualified to testify as an expert and that the testimony is reliable. Reliability is shown only where the testimony is based on sufficient facts or data and is the product of generally accepted principles and methods. Qualified experts in this area have frequently been accepted as experts in our federal district courts.

Counsel in jail suicide cases seek expert consultants and witnesses whose qualifications and experience will render their opinions valuable and whose testimony, if necessary, will be deemed admissible under prevailing court standards. Among the critical considerations are:

1. *Background and Experience*

In determining whether an expert possesses the required background and experience, council will consider the expert's education, particularly in the mental health professions, teaching, and publications in relevant areas, as well as specialized training and experience in the areas of individual and municipal liability that are directly pertinent to the issues raised in a particular case. The experience should include specialized training in and knowledge of pertinent policy issues, research, scholarship, and applicable legal principles. Further, and critically, the expert should be familiar with applicable issues of the training, supervision, and monitoring of prison mental health providers to determine whether accepted practices and protocols have been followed in a particular case. Experts in jail suicide cases generally evaluate complex mental health issues, related medical concerns, and the use of prescribed medications. Experts who possess medical degrees in psychiatry are frequently considered the most qualified and effective.

2. *Reliability of Opinions*

The requisite education and experience of a proposed professional do not in and of itself render that person an "expert" in the areas of jail suicide cases. The expert must know how to evaluate the facts and record of a case in a manner that supports the basis for the opinions he or she renders in the case. The expert must cite research, empirical data, and/or relevant scholarship to support any findings, and provide specific citations to the record (and not extract facts selectively and out of context).

In short, an expert must demonstrate compliance with the Daubert standards: There must be a showing that the expert's theory can be (or has been) tested by experts in the field, that it has been subject to peer review; there should be an acknowledgment of the known or potential rate of error in the theory, and whether the theory is generally accepted in the relevant community. Separately, there must be a showing of the "fit" that is required of any expert testimony, that it is relevant to the issues to be decided in the case. Finally, as an expert's testimony on issues of law are inadmissible, any opinion must not contain an impermissible legal conclusion which improperly intrude upon the exclusive province of the court.

3. *Ability to Communicate*

There is another important consideration in the choice of an expert—the ability of the individual to communicate effectively with counsel and, importantly, before the judge or jury. An expert should communicate simply, succinctly, and in a manner that does not make it appear that the expert is "talking down" to the judge or jury. When a technical term is used, the witness should explain the meaning of the term in everyday language (or, better still, avoid the unnecessary use of technical terms).

—Paul Messing

Kairys Rudovsky Messing Feinberg & Lin, LLP, 718 Arch Street, Suite 501S, Philadelphia, PA 19106

13. JESUS EDUARDO ARIAS, CERRITOS, CALIFORNIA

What are the factors that you weigh in choosing an expert to work on your case?

Experience and credentials on the field of expertise. (Solid Background) "Qualification"

Experience in prior testimony given for similar-type cases. Both in depositions and at trial—"Litigation Experience"

"Personality." The type of person who could explain to the jury the nature and context of his opinions but in a way that ANYONE can understand it. With inherent authority on the field by way of his experience, but with humble ability to talk to jury not in a condescending manner, but rather in an explanatory manner. An expert's job is to aid the trier of fact, not lecture him or her or impress him or her or even worse, confuse him or her.

That is reasonable in his fees. And working conditions. Responsible with writing reports, etc. Available to talk to or phone call or email to discuss the matter. In short, a professional.

Are any or all factors noted in Rule 702 or any other factors, given special weight?

In my practice, the personality has a special weight. If the person is a brilliant expert science type person, however has serious problems communicating and explaining the basis and core of his opinions, I would rather look for another expert. Perhaps not so brilliant in the field but experienced enough with good communication skills to relate to the jury and explain the basis for his opinions better.

—Jesus Eduardo Arias Esq. LL.M.
18000 Studebaker Rd. 700, Cerritos, CA 90703

14. NADERH ELRABADI, CHICAGO, ILLINOIS

The use of experts is instrumental in tying together causation, damages, and future loss. For the experience related to correctional centers, it is beneficial to navigate with an expert, since I have an obligation to my client to prove damages and then explain to the judge or jury the intricacies of an issue, policies, and procedures. The use of the expert as a plaintiff is to educate the jury from the perspective of an impartial evaluator. We rely on experts to show that the party does not sway their opinions that they represent. Thus, the expert must have expertise in evaluating defense and plaintiff cases. This gives the jury the ability to judge the credibility of the witness.

—Nader H. Elrabadi
ELRABADI LAW, 22 W. Washington Street, Suite 1500, Chicago, IL 60602

15. CHRISTOPHER GRABAREK, CROWN POINT, INDIANA

Arrogance is an indicator that the expert will not be likable or understandable. Their inflated egos encourage them to believe that the jurors should be honored to be in their presence. Most experts are also difficult to work with. Even though it is subconscious, they put their interest first. Believe it or not, it is difficult to find experts who care. I have now tried, as lead counsel, over ninety jury trials. I have an unorthodox approach: I typically do not call any witnesses. That way, I can control everything, and I do not worry about my expert agreeing with opposing counsel. As mentioned, I have been subject to countless hacks. These days, I develop points upon which my opponent experts, and all my opponent's witnesses, will agree with me. I work hard to determine when to go— with every witness. As such, if the witness disagrees with me, I demonstrate to the jury that they are not credible. And nothing goes further with the jury than credibility.

Over the years, I learned that jury duty is anathema for most of our citizens, which is the reason they strive to avoid it. When the potential jurors arrive at the courthouse the first day, they are often bitter and, at times, even hostile. They are forced to miss work and be away from their families. They blame the lawyers for being issued the summons which orders the potential jurors to appear at the courthouse.

In essence, their egos cause some expert witnesses to be oblivious to one of the most fundamental and important aspects of a jury trial. That is, the jury, exclusively, makes the determination of the outcome of the trial. Not the judge, not any of the lawyers, and not any of the insurance adjusters. Therefore, the much greater emphasis should be placed on the jury. Many lawyers disregard the value of providing the jury with an understanding of the complicated and technical issues. To prevail at trial, it is imperative that the jury comprehend complicated and technical issues.

Using expert witness's testimony, the jury can acquire the understanding of complex and technical issues. The burden for this ultimately rests with the lawyer. It is imperative that the lawyer devote significant time and energy into acquiring an understanding of the expert's subject matter. At the end of the day, it is the lawyer's obligation to ensure that the jury comprehends the expert testimony. If the expert's testimony is not comprehended by the jury, then the testimony will result in confusion and potentially frustration by the jurors.

Notwithstanding the attitudes of some expert witnesses, his/her role is not to demonstrate his/her brilliance and display his/her sophistication at every conceivable situation. For most jurors, conceit and demonstrations of erudition are indicators that the expert witness feels a sense of superiority to the jury. During a jury trial, being effete is not an attribute. Too often, the expert witness's demeanor and attitude is aloof and patronizing. If possible, the expert witness conduct himself/herself in a manner that is not pretentious. Furthermore, if the expert can display empathy for the jurors, then the expert's ability to connect with the jury will be greatly enhanced. Remember, the juror's attendance has been compelled.

It is appperative that the expert articulates the concepts in comprehensible language rather than in technical and/or abstruse scientific terms. For the jury to understand the expert, it is essential that the expert witness use commonly understood, everyday language. Speaking in plain English has tremendous value in many respects. Indeed, it helps foster a connection with the jury. In this regard, the expert witness, while testifying, should look at the jury and speak directly to the jury. This establishes a connection with the jury.

—Christopher Grabarek
    Johnson and Bell, 1041 Broadway, Crown Point, IN 46307

16. JOHN RAY III, CHICAGO, ILLINOIS

In assessing experts, the most important factor that I consider is his or her relatability to the jury. I try to determine who I believe will be able to establish a connection with the jurors, based on his or her professional and personal connection to the local community, the depth of his or her experience and knowledge within that community, and his or her personality. Trust in and, therefore, deference to the opinion of an expert is formed by how well an expert can connect, so I assess the strength of their connections to the people who will be asked to consider his or her testimony.

But, before getting to a jury, a judge is often asked (by the opposing party) to determine whether an expert has sufficient basis for his or her testimony, and under Rue 702, I have found that the most critical assessments by judges lie in Rule 702(b) and (d), with emphasis on 702(d). Establishing the factual predicate of the opinion is important, but much of that work is often performed in conjunction with the attorneys in the case. The strength of an expert to a court as the gatekeeper lies in his or her ability to take the facts developed and apply whatever scientific or technical principles, incorporating those facts into a reasoned report and opinion.

—John H. Ray, III
   Ray & Counsel, P.C.—New York/Chicago/Boston, 10044
      South Leavitt Street, Chicago, IL 60643

17. CHRISTOPHER S. MORRIS, SAN DIEGO, CALIFORNIA

When looking for an expert, I consider several factors. First, I like my expert to be a practitioner in the field at issue. The jury often views experts that have long since removed themselves from the day-to-day activities as simply a "hired gun." I will also ask for their prior testimony on the issues at hand to ensure that they have not taken an opposite position in the past. Finally, I like my experts to put me to the test. I want my theories to be tested and bandied about. I like it when an expert tells me that they cannot testify to something because it shows to me that they believe the things they are willing to testify.

—Christopher S. Morris
   Morris Law Firm, APC, 501 West Broadway, Suite 1480,
      San Diego, CA 92101

18. HERBERT TERRELL, MCDONALD, PENNSYLVANIA

I did not consider to any extent the Rule 702 requirements. I rather focused upon the expert's background and subject matter expertise. I was attracted to you because of a referral wherein I was told you had written extensively about detainee/inmate co-occurring disability.

—Herbert A. Terrell, Esquire
   201 Liberty Street, McDonald, PA 15057

19. TREY YARBROUGH, TYLER, TEXAS

My starting point for the selection of an expert in federal court suicide-related cases is, of course, Rule 702 and the requirements set forth therein. That being a given, the factors I consider as an attorney selecting an expert in a jail (or other incarceration) suicide-related case include the following:

1. The expert's depth of education and experience in psychiatry
2. The expert's depth of hands-on experience and knowledge in jail and/or prison management, supervision, and oversight
3. The expert's depth of knowledge with respect to national and statewide standards and protocols relative to jail/prison management, supervision, and oversight
4. The expert's experience in testifying in such cases, whether by deposition or trial
5. Based on initial interviews and history with other attorneys, the expert's perceived ability to communicate and present well to a jury with respect to a subject matter that is very foreign to most laypersons
6. Based on the expert's past record and through the interview process, the expert's seeming commitment to a meticulous and thorough investigation and analysis of the case facts and documentation
7. Based on the interview process and history with other attorneys, the expert's perceived demeanor with respect to credibility, frankness, and transparency

8. Based on the interview process and history with other attorneys, the expert's commitment to meeting court-ordered deadlines, and the expert's responsiveness to the needs of the case and the attorney

—*Trey Yarbrough*

Yarbrough Wilcox, PLLC, 100 E. Ferguson St., Suite 1015 Tyler, TX 75702

ACKNOWLEDGMENTS

It has been a privilege to share my ideas and professional expertise on the prevention and litigation aspects of suicide in jails and prisons. Once I committed to writing the book, not an easy task, I was able to marshal encouragement and support from many people and resources, some seen and some unseen.

I want to thank Mary Lou Reid of Los Angeles, my Book Coach, who meticulously and diligently enabled me to conceptualize the book and then obsessively guided me at every step of the way. Mary Lou is a unique taskmaster who brought out the best in my writing in her quiet manner.

My initial readers included Sandra Kardinal, a good family friend, and Abraham Joseph, MD, Anesthesiology and Critical Care Specialist (Armed Forces Medical Services, India) and M. V. Pillai, MD, Clinical Professor of Oncology, Thomas Jefferson University, Philadelphia, both my medical school classmates. They carefully read the early iterations of the first few chapters and provided valuable direction and advice. Later, Palpu Hazel, MD, a psychiatrist, read a few chapters and advised me on the flow of ideas and readability. In this context, I want to thank my medical school classmates and friends, particularly K. Ravindran, MD, DCH,

Jaya Ramanathan, MD, C. Thomas, MS, FRCS; M. B. Nair, MS; N.K. Ponnamma, MD; Annamma Salam, MD; S. Venugopal, MS, FACS; and Viji Vellody, MD, who encouraged and supported my writing.

As the writing progressed, I was able to rely on the expertise and wisdom of Fred Rottnek, MD, Professor of Family Medicine at St. Louis University School of Medicine, an eminent correctional health-care practitioner and expert consultant. In addition, I want to thank Richard Lichten, a jail and police expert who contributed a great deal to the book's contents. Finally, my gratitude extends to Percy Menzies, M. Pharm, a lifelong friend and a source of personal inspiration who directed me to Dr. Rottnek.

Encouragement for my authorship came from a famous author, Jack Canfield, of *Chicken Soup for the Soul*, who carefully read the first five chapters. I express my gratitude to him for his approval of my writing.

I thank Tyler Alexander, a research attorney at Casetext .com, a legal database, who answered every question about legal source documents, Federal and Supreme Court cases included in various chapters. Also, I thank two legal consultants who offered valuable suggestions and recommendations on legal issues addressed in the book.

I thank the expert work by Michele DeFilippo, Ronda Rawlins, and Anita Salzberg (editor) of 1106 Design that produced the final product in book form.

I express my deepest gratitude to Ruthann Harper, my office manager, who for over forty years has put up with me, typed, and edited all the cases in which I was involved. She provided valuable insights, placing herself as a juror while reading my

Rule 26 reports. In addition, she typed this entire manuscript and provided valuable editorial input.

Roger Moore, who chauffeured me to jails, prisons, and courts during the last five years, listened to my case stories, and shared occasional wisdom as a layperson.

I want to thank my patients, mental health professionals, correctional officers, administrators, attorneys, judges, and families I have encountered from whom I drew strength to pursue my interest on the subject.

I thank my family, including Sheeba Daniel-Crotty, PhD, Steven Crotty, MD, Mariam Stevens, MD, and Tyler Stevens, MD, for their discussions on the subject and my five lovely grandchildren. Tyler provided extensive editorial assistance for all chapters. Benjamin Crotty, now a USC student, did basic research on prisoner statistics and institutions. My gratitude extends to my parents, Dr. A. D. Easo and Mrs. Kunjamma, a teacher who instilled in me that you serve others with your words and deeds. I thank my sisters, Prof. Sally Cherian and Mrs. Shirly Thomas (India).

Finally, I am indebted to my beloved life partner and wife Molly Daniel, who from day one has been my unwavering support and source of strength as I have pursued this project.

—Anasseril E. Daniel, MD

INDEX

ABOUT THE AUTHOR

orensic psychiatrist Anasseril E. Daniel, MD, has devoted
the last twenty years of his professional life to correctional
mental health and psychiatry. Dr. Daniel has consulted with
attorneys, testified in court, and authored peer-reviewed articles on inmate suicide risk identification and prevention, as
well as risk management strategies relating to suicide. Along
with seven distinguished suicide researchers and clinicians
from Europe, Canada, Australia, and the United States, he
coauthored the World Health Organization (WHO) Resource
Guide: "Preventing Suicide in Jails and Prisons" (2007). Dr.
Daniel is Adjunct Professor of Psychiatry at the University of
Missouri School of Medicine.

From 1984 to 1991 Dr. Daniel was the executive director of
Mid-Missouri Mental Center in Columbia, Missouri. Between
2001 and 2007, he worked as the Director of Psychiatric
Services for the Missouri Department of Corrections. During
his directorship, he developed a keen interest in suicide and
studied the pattern of suicide in the Missouri Department of
Corrections between 1992 and 2001. He assisted in developing suicide prevention policies and procedures for the Boone

County Jail in Columbia, Missouri, and for the Missouri Department of Corrections.

Dr. Daniel has provided direct psychiatric services to mentally ill suicidal inmates and worked with correctional officers who provide one-on-one supervision. He is passionate about preventing suicides in jails and prisons and has conducted seminars and in-service training on suicide prevention and interventional strategies for correctional mental health and custodial staff. Dr. Daniel has also created a training module for correctional officers.

Through his research, studies, and practice, Dr. Daniel established himself as an expert on suicide in jails and prisons. A sought-after expert consultant and witness in suicide-related lawsuits, he has provided expert consultations to attorneys in seventy-five suicide-related litigations across the United States and testified by deposition and in jury trials. He has helped attorneys reach case settlements and/or defend their clients. He continues to practice as an expert consultant and witness in Columbia, Missouri.

An online educational course titled, "Prevent Suicide in Jails and Prisons: Avoid Lawsuits" for correctional officials and mental health professionals will be available soon. As an educator, trainer and speaker, Dr. Daniel will be available to speak on suicide prevention in jails and prisons.

For more information visit
www.PrisonSuicideExpertWitness.com
Contact: aedaniel@aol.com, anasserildaniel@gmail.com

www.ingramcontent.com/pod-product-compliance
Lightning Source LLC
Chambersburg PA
CBHW070826110726
47973CB00029B/277/J